NURSING HISTORY REVIEW

OFFICIAL JOURNAL OF THE AMERICAN ASSOCIATION FOR THE HISTORY OF NURSING
1994 • Volume 2
University of Pennsylvania Press

CONTENTS

Volume 2 1994

Nursing History Review

Nursing History Review is published annually for the American Association for the History of Nursing, Inc., by the University of Pennsylvania Press.

International Standard Serial Number ISSN 1062-8061
International Standard Book Number ISBN 0-8122-1451-X (Volume 2)
Printed in the United States of America

All inquiries concerning subscriptions or advertising should be sent to:

Marketing Department
University of Pennsylvania Press
418 Service Drive
Philadelphia, Pa. 19104-6097
Attention: Subscription Manager

Yearly subscription rates are: $35.00, individuals; $50.00, institutions and libraries.

Members of the American Association for the History of Nursing, Inc. (AAHN) receive *Nursing History Review* on payment of $60.00 annual membership dues. Applications and other correspondence relating to AAHN membership should be directed to:

Dr. Rosemary McCarthy, Executive Director
American Association for the History of Nursing, Inc.
P.O. Box 90803
Washington, D.C. 20090-0803

Please direct all submissions and editorial correspondence to:

Joan E. Lynaugh, Editor
Nursing History Review
University of Pennsylvania
420 Guardian Drive, Room 307
Philadelphia, Pa. 19104-6096

EDITORIAL

The contributors are rushing to put the finishing touches on their articles while we, here in *NHR*'s editorial office, assemble the completed manuscript, photographs, drawings, and other material to send to Penn Press. I keep recalling the refrain on the last page of A. A. Milne's *Now We Are Six*, which begins, "When I was One I had just begun. When I was Two I was nearly new."* With just two volumes *Nursing History Review* is truly "nearly new." But the range and quality of historical scholarship in our field is affirmed by the articles and reviews you will find again this year. I commend them to you.

Read Diane Hamilton and Victoria Slater as they dissect the intellectual and philosophical foundations of modern nursing—while Sandra Lewenson and Ruth Malone assess the social and political strategies and struggles of professionalizing women. Susan Smith finds entirely new historical territory in the public health history of the American South, while Linda Walsh analyzes the real lives of midwives in urban practice in a northern American city. Quincealea Brunk restores to our collective memory the nineteenth-century Civil War nurses who invented nursing as we came to know it. Irene Poplin seeks out rare sources to explain the symbolic and practical meaning behind nurses' traditional garb.

With this issue we begin what we hope will become a pattern of publishing scholarship from the worldwide community of historians interested in nursing. Marianne Tallberg generously helped us gain access to her excellent paper on eighteenth- and nineteenth-century health care in Finland. Barbara Brush and Meryn Stuart inaugurate our feature called "Doing the Work of History" as they discuss the complexities of internationally focused historical research on women. We hope to attract more such papers for this new methodology section to stimulate a dialogue on the intellectual and technical problems of "doing history" in our many-faceted field.

Historians have contributed eleven scholarly book reviews for this issue. We believe book reviews to be a service to all peoples of our historical community: researchers, students, educators, consumers of good history, and, of course, the authors of the reviewed books. We hope you concur; please share your opinions with us.

*A. A. Milne, *Now We Are Six* (New York: E. P. Dutton and Co., 1927).

We are already at work on the next issue—becoming "Three." To be the best possible vehicle for historical research, we need responses from our readers. Let us know how you feel about the *Review*—its direction, its articles, its look. This is a great time for the history of nursing. Be a part of it.

Joan E. Lynaugh
Center for the Study of the History of Nursing
University of Pennsylvania

Editor's note:

The following acknowledgment note to Carol Helmstadter's "Old Nurses and New" was inadvertently omitted from the last volume of *Nursing History Review:*

I am indebted to the Social Science and Humanities Research Council of Canada, which provided the funding for the research project of which this article is a part, and to the Ontario Nurses' Association for their generosity in allowing me time to write it.

Constructing the Mind of Nursing

DIANE HAMILTON
School of Nursing
University of Rochester

Revisionist historical scholars have lately expanded the explanations of nursing's conception beyond "the great woman theory" of Nightingale's genius to suggest that American nursing's roots emanate from a blending of the ideology of domesticity with that of medical science (O'Brien 1987; Lynaugh and Fagin 1988); that nursing is a story of women workers' rationalizing the service industry (Melosh 1982); that nursing is the product of a group of enlightened leaders intent on reform and professionalization (Christy 1969); that nursing developed from the growth of paternalistic hospitals eager to manipulate females and to profit from nurses' work (Ashley 1976); that nursing emerged from interacting social and economic needs related to the care of the ill (Rosenberg 1987); that nursing became visible when philanthropic women and physicians demanded that hospitals employ "lady" nurses (Mottus 1981); and that nursing gained its social and moral justification from its obligation to care (Reverby 1987).[1] Historical inquiry fuels an interpretive argument about the past; each perspective generates new insights to and another link in the great chain of explanation and understanding of nursing's history. At the same time we are reminded of unanswered, tantalizing questions.

One genre of unasked questions concerns the ideas on which nurses built their work. What could we discover by conceptualizing nurses' *thinking* as the object of historical research? What were the thoughts and the thinking patterns of the leaders who designed nursing as a vocation for

Nursing History Review 2 (1994): 3–28.

women? And what are the epistemological and ontological assumptions rooted in the history of nurses' thinking?

We know that during the nineteenth century nursing began to distinguish itself from other groups, to organize its activities, and to seek credibility and legitimacy within society. The nurse inventors believed that nurses offered an esoteric service to the public based on some special conception of knowledge. As emerging professionals, nurses professed "to know." Yet the intellectual terrain of nursing remains unexplored. While giving Florence Nightingale credit as nursing's first "theorist," many writers seem to assume that "nursing theory and knowledge development have a short history."[2] This leaves us with a mental picture of a great wasteland of unthinking nurses stretching from Nightingale to mid-twentieth-century nurse thinkers such as Hildegarde Peplau, Faye G. Abdellah, and Ernestine Weidenbach. The apex of thinking, according to this ahistorical view, occurs with the nurse theorists of the late twentieth century. This notion that sophisticated thinking and theorizing began only recently presumes that "modern" ideas are innately superior to earlier ones. It denies that the nurse inventors and nurses who followed were bright, articulate women. These women directed health and illness-related institutions, and they were fully capable of generating concepts, ideas, and meanings. To view late-twentieth-century nursing knowledge as "new" denies the probability that ideas emigrated and immigrated over multiple generations of nurses and nurse-institutions in a social context that perpetually sculpted ideas and thinking.

This article reexamines and reflects on a small "thought collective" (a term I explain below) of nurses, Lillian Wald, Annie Goodrich, and Lavinia Dock. In it I argue that the institution of nursing includes an intellectual history as much as an economic, social, and a political one. Moreover, I will show that, while Wald, Goodrich, and Dock believed their ideas to be "modern" and secular, their conceptualization of nursing rested on religious and spiritual ideas of earlier eras. From these ideas, they selected compassion to be one of the basic guiding principles and virtues of nursing.

Toward the end of the nineteenth century, an amalgam of many ideas coalesced to transform nursing from a servile occupation into a paid vocation. The training school movement, from a slow beginning in the midcentury, began to flourish—growing from thirty-five schools in 1890 to 432 schools by the close of the century. Although nursing leaders at the World's Fair in Chicago in 1893 protested against the overwhelming lack of uniformity of instruction in schools of nursing, successful training programs,

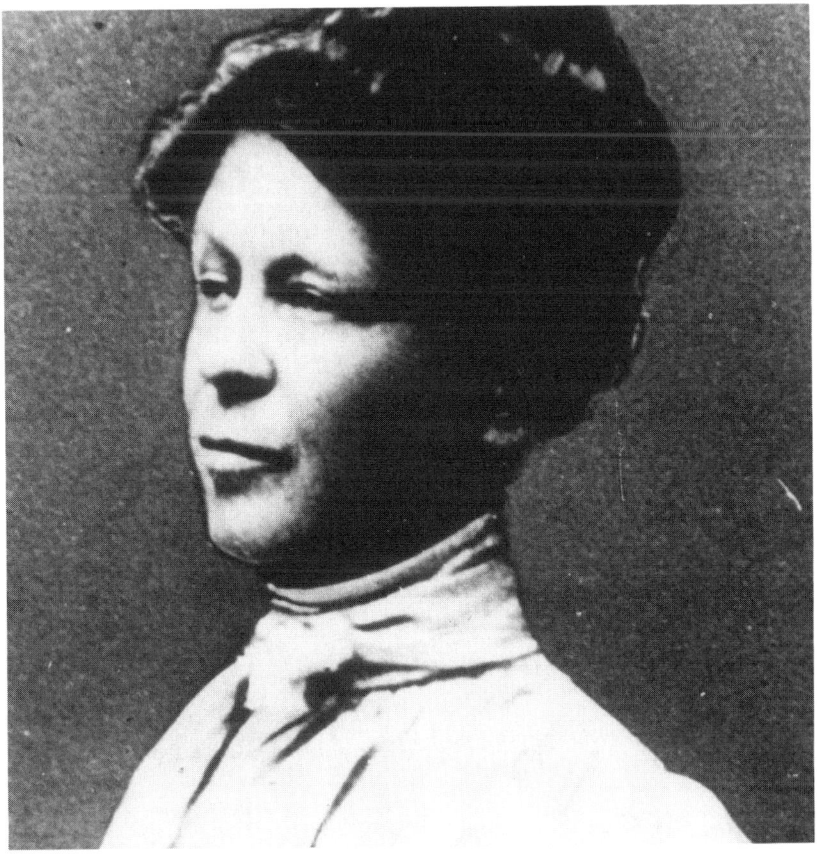

Lavinia L. Dock. (Courtesy of the Center for the Study of the History of Nursing)

boasting of both educational standards and strong nursing leadership, were established at several teaching hospitals, including The Johns Hopkins, Bellevue, Boston City, Massachusetts General, New York Hospital, and Connecticut Training School at the New Haven Hospital. Moreover, the American Society of Superintendents of Training Schools for Nurses, later called the National League for Nursing Education, had organized in 1894, and the Nurses' Associated Alumnae of the United States and Canada, which became the American Nurses' Association, formed two years later.[3]

This flurry of organizing, in retrospect, was not surprising. Historians generally agree that in the late nineteenth century, Americans from every class organized, usually by occupation, in an effort to adapt to a changing

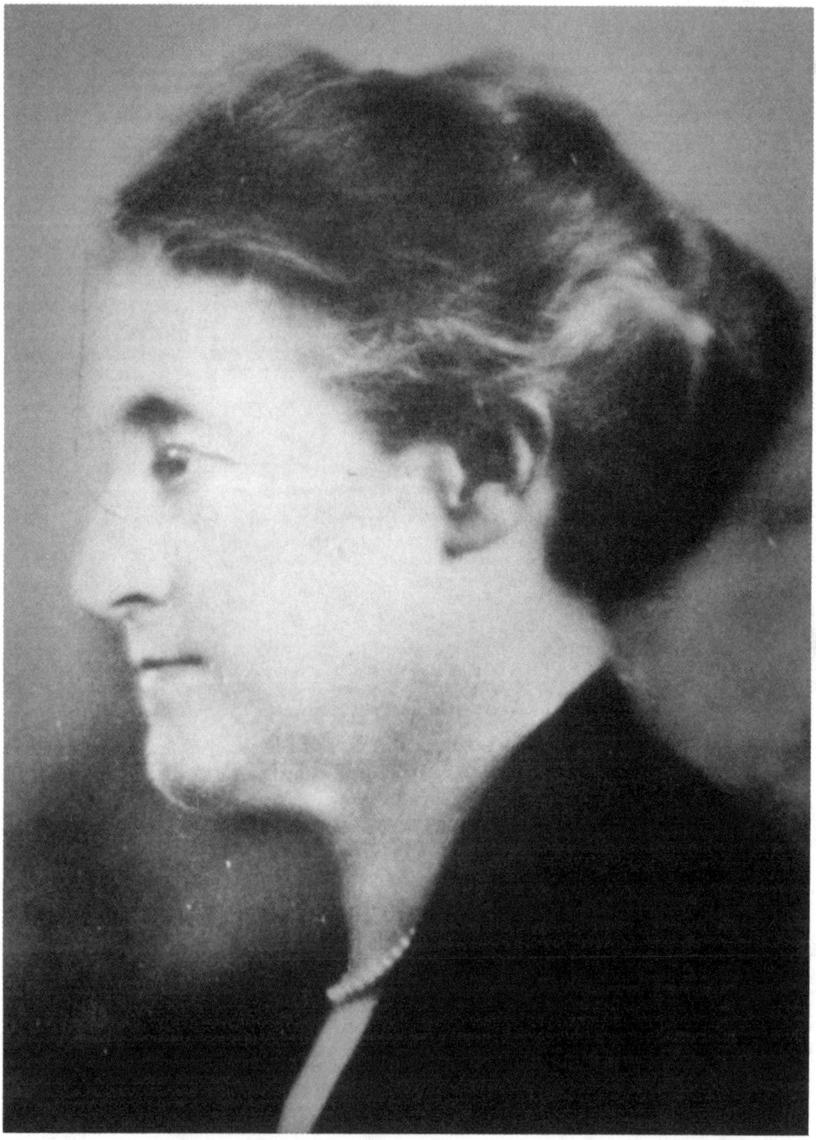

Annie W. Goodrich. (Courtesy of the Center for the Study of the History of Nursing)

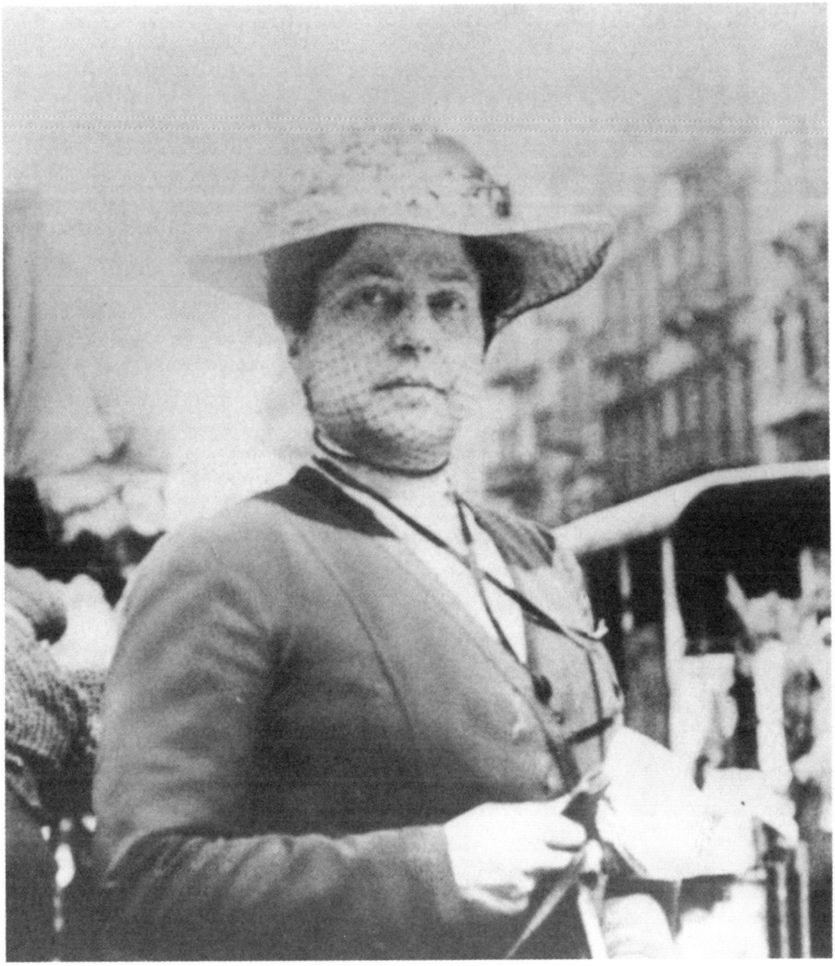

Lillian D. Wald. (Courtesy of the Visiting Nurse Service of New York)

society and economy.[4] The professions, in general, shifted their intellectual orientation from an individualistic and voluntary approach to a collective one in order to function more effectively and thus obtain status, legitimacy, and profit. Nurses, following the footsteps of the more established professions, such as medicine and law, began to form organizations, to standardize educational requirements, to establish journals, and to persuade state legislatures to pass registration and licensing laws.

Intellectual History: Unearth the Thinking

Nurse inventors needed an intellectual framework to guide their process of legitimizing nursing. To solidify the concept "nurse," to construct the phenomenon called "professional nursing," to fashion the boundaries of rightness and wrongness of nurse behavior, and to effectively negotiate acceptance of the validity of the trained nurse necessitated both competing ideas and some degree of "sameness of thinking" among the nurse inventors. Yet the exact nature of the nurse inventors' intellectual schema for constructing the "mind of nursing" remains unarticulated.

Ian Hacking, analyzing the relationship between reality and labels, called this legitimating process "making people up" and suggested that the proliferation of labels in the nineteenth century engendered more kinds of people than ever before.[5] As new institutions created new labels, people came forward to accept the labels and to construct their lives accordingly. While nursing had always been part of women's "natural" work, by mid-century nursing had evolved into an occupation with women willing to perform the work for wages, to organize nursing's structure and function, and to profess ideas about nursing in the marketplace.

As new ideas emerge, they carry the marks of their social origins. Classifications, logical thinking, and guiding metaphors are socially constructed, linking ideas and cognition to political, economic, and social problems. What is considered of value or "true" varies across time, for society's perspective is determined by dominant opinions and directed perceptions, popularly labeled the dominant "paradigm" (Kuhn 1962) or "thought style" (Fleck 1979). And although thought styles function as a prism in which reality is refracted, individuals, needing to build a meaningful world, choose from the thought style's smorgasbord of ideas through the groups in which they live. According to philosopher Ludwig Fleck (1979), a group of persons, working and exchanging ideas within institutions, constitutes a thought collective.[6] Thus, thought collectives, functioning within the era's thought style, become the distributors and brokers of institutions' ideas.[7]

Of course, the effect of accepting both the individual and the social context as sculptors of ideas highlights the thorny issue of the relationship between the individual mind and social influences on cognition, between the subjective perceptions and social context, and between the subjective (inside) and the objective (outside) reality of the lived human experience.[8] These dilemmas cannot be ignored by historians studying thinking as a historical event. As historian Dominick LaCapra pointed out, while the social context may, in part, explain how social problems influence the origin of ideas, the social context may neither directly *cause* the ideas nor illucidate the authors' intentions or *meaning* of the ideas.[9] Describing an idea's origin and understanding the meaning of authors' thinking are different. To disclose meaning and offer interpretation, the historian must search for the relationship between the author's intentions and the text, the relationship between the author's life and the text, and the interaction between the culture and its institution and the text, while maintaining the awareness that these relationships will include multiple forms of tensions, incongruities, and contradictions. A good historical interpretation of ideas does not simply impose coherence on what seem to be "scattered" thoughts, but rather stimulates further investigation into seemingly incompatible ideas and beliefs.

An analysis of nurse inventors' thinking cannot suggest that their ideas simply mirrored the pragmatist, the progressive, or the populist thoughts of the historical era that midwived nursing. The notions of nursing are strongly influenced by, but not necessarily caused by, intellectual trends. Nursing was not discovered as a completed product, but rather was constructed by a multitude of persons, in multiple settings, and within more than one context.

Nursing history is not only a story of what happened to whom and when; it is also an analysis of who we are, why we think the way we do, and how the ideas of "what nursing *should* be" and "what nursing is" changed over time. In the process of envisioning and bonding to the identity, the thinking, and the mission of nursing, the nurse inventors fashioned a core of ideas within their social context. They selected ideas that seemed good and true and right for nursing practice, for society, and, maybe more importantly, for themselves. Nursing foremothers such as Lillian Wald, Isabel Hampton Robb, Lavinia Dock, Annie Goodrich, Lillian Clayton, Mary Lent, Ella Crandall, Mary Gardner, Adelaide Nutting, Sophia Palmer, Isabel McIsaac, Mary E. P. Davis, and Louise Darche engaged in, and in many ways formulated, the precedent of "nurse thinking and nursing practice" during what historian Teresa Christy called "the fateful decade" (1890–1900).[10]

The Fateful Decade

By 1890, just a hundred years after the founding of the Republic, the American promise of egalitarian life was becoming an illusion. The extremes of wealth and poverty were as great as those in the Old World. The structure of American industry had changed dramatically from widespread small-town shopkeeping into centralized, large-scale manufacturing, with national market corporations in a few cities. Small towns shrank in political and economic significance while the complexity and density of industrial and seaport cities increased, with millions of immigrants crowding into the slums of American cities, constituting a proletariat that was not only impoverished but alien.

Despite these social and economic threats to continuity, America was in a hurry to be great. Americans had convinced themselves that their country was predestined for superiority by accepting the doctrine of social Darwinism that promised success to the strong and envisioned progress as an ever accelerating movement. That freedom and democracy would eventually create a pure, rational society seemed obvious to Americans. Moreover, it seemed self-evident that the accumulation of knowledge would catapult society into a promising future. The last decade of the nineteenth century did produce a large body of new thinking, such as James's *Psychology;* Veblen's *Theory of the Leisure Class;* Wine's *Report on Crime and Pauperism;* Boas's *Development of the Culture of Northwest America;* and Dewey's *The School and Society.* But despite idealistic attitudes and an accumulation of knowledge, utopia always seemed just around the corner. As Henry Commager noted, "never had men known so many facts and been masters of so few principles."[11]

Surrounded by the often dismal conditions of a shifting society, Americans could not deny the physical and spiritual reality of the disenfranchised poor. As historian Robert Wiebe notes, late-nineteenth-century America had to acknowledge that society had lost its core and sense of community. As this sobering awareness permeated society, the crises of the communities surfaced as a syndrome that included lack of confidence in the powers of the community, anxiety about self-determination, a search for order, and an enthusiasm for reform.[12]

Harsh urban realities demanded reform. With labor rioting, child mortality rates increasing, and diseases like tuberculosis and syphilis running rampant across class lines, reformers approached the problems with a mood of excited urgency. While some reformers reordered government, child labor laws, or prisons, others entered the city slums to live among the poor. Settlement houses, as outposts of education and culture within depraved cities, were intended to bridge the gulf between the classes, to lessen suspicion and hostility between diverse cultural groups, and to do more than just "hand out" charity. The educated, the cultured, and the privileged "settled" among the poor in order to, as Jane Addams described the movement, "equalize opportunity," not from a motive of philanthropy nor benevolence but from a "sense of humanity."[13]

As a comprehensive institution within the communities, the settlement house, which Jane Addams compared to a university, stood for the application of knowledge, as opposed to research; for emotion and humanity, in contrast to intellectualization; and for equalizing life experiences and opportunities among classes. One natural link to this civic humanism was the public health movement, which, as all nurses know, capitalized on visiting nurses. Equalizing opportunity for the poor and dedication to social welfare in the broadest sense had to include sanitation, hygiene, and regulation of the environments that produced disease. Middle-class reformers found it difficult to enlighten the mind and the spirit without feeding, clothing, sheltering, and caring for the body. Thus, the public health reformers found an easy alliance between the institutions of visiting nurses and settlement houses. The public health movement, designed to be broad in scope, concerned itself with almost every aspect of life: the promotion of health, the prevention of disease, and the maintenance of a standard of living necessary for health. The settlement house movement juxtaposed with the public health movement addressed human welfare in the very broadest sense.[14]

Women, as keepers of the culture's mores, played a major role in these humanistic civic movements. For many of the women serving the settlement house cause, the movement offered opportunities for companionship, intimacy, and self-development, and a purpose for their life. With few employment opportunities open to them, settlement houses became for women a viable option, enabling them to live and work interdependently. Historian William O'Neill coined the phrase "social feminism" as an explanation for women's strong dedication to ideas of social justice and solidarity, while Ellen Lagemann suggests that women's "natural" maternal instinct obligated them to make America a kinder place. Barbara Welter argued that these women moved into the corrupt and unjust cities to transfer the cultural assumptions of women's innate piety, purity, and domesticity onto the urban landscape. Caroll Smith-Rosenberg labeled the woman associated with the settlement house movement "the New Woman," in that she was unmarried, rejected social conventions, and asserted her right to visible power and a public voice. Susan Armeny argued that an older complex of attitudes, called the "sanitary ideal," which loathed individualism and waste but admired order and discipline, provided the motivation and sustaining energy of the settlement house women.[15]

The society of the "fateful decade" resonated to an anxious but hopeful rhythm in which ideas of reform, progress, democracy, idealism, good women, and justice harmonized. Cultural presumptions of the nineteenth century imbued the reformers with a belief that social progress brought democracy and that personal independence conferred personhood and citizenship. They assumed that nothing was beyond their power because they believed that social, economic, and political equity would eventually lead to a less chaotic and fragmented world capable of human perfectability.

A Nursing Thought Collective

Ideas of reform, progress, womanhood, justice, and the public's health influenced, enabled, and restricted the nurse inventors' possibilities of thought and focused the mental lens through which they experienced and interpreted reality. The institutions in which the nurse inventors worked and lived provided a second layer of framing. Hospitals, settlement houses, and instructive nursing associations, each with distinctive cultures and politics, provided different institutional contexts for nursing ideas. Moreover, each nurse inventor had personal motivations that influenced her thinking. Thus, society, institutions, and personhood homogenized to create complex contexts in which nurse inventors shaped nursing, created the classification of "trained nurse," and attempted to sculpt reality to validate their ideal.

Although the list of eminent nursing inventors is lengthy, three well-known nurses seem to form a coterie of thinkers.[16] Born within the same decade, their paths crossed at Henry Street Settlement House in New York City, an institution that became agent and counteragent for the ideas that they hoped to broker. Lillian Wald, Lavinia Dock, and Annie Goodrich were very different women whose life journeys became indelibly interconnected, yet their ideas, beliefs, and classifications coalesced to form a foundation for generations of nurses who followed. Wald, Dock, and Goodrich believed they represented a new enlightened era for nursing. And, when thinkers agree that their present day is like no other period, and that a great gulf divides them from the past, philosopher Ludwig Fleck suggests that a thought collective is identifiable.[17] Clearly, Wald, Dock, and Goodrich set themselves apart and relished "modern" nursing's distinctiveness from previous eras of nursing.

Lavinia Dock, addressing the Nurses' Associated Alumnae in 1907, remarked that ancient nursing represented crude ministrations of healing, but that "modern" nursing had finally grasped the essential idea that health was related to social responsibility, social progress, and moral obligation.[18] Dock held that "modern" nursing must be a force in reversing the pathology of human misery and in triumphantly unifying mankind through the spirit of progress. The notion of progress also appealed to Goodrich, who suggested that the "promise of the period upon which nursing has now entered" was self-evident, with the "ills to which man was prey for centuries tracked down and destroyed."[19] Modern nursing was ordained to participate in rearranging life and in transforming society to greater heights. Remarking that "nursing is no longer the handmaiden of the physician, the official wife of medicine, nor the younger sister of the medical family," Wald promoted an independent nursing profession—one that would transfuse hope to the miserable experiences of the masses.[20] And as authors of classic texts, these women, individually and collectively, hoped that their gospels would influence a great awakening within nursing, with individual nurses collectively responsible for the birth of civic righteousness and for the transformation of a troubled society.[21]

Born in the mid-1880s into upper-middle-class families, Dock (1858–1956), Wald (1867–1940), and Goodrich (1866–1955) describe a restlessness in their early lives. Their writings exude a longing to find an opportunity for intellectual self-fulfillment and to have an autonomous role outside their nuclear families. From a practical viewpoint, both Dock and Goodrich reluctantly admitted that their families' financial reversals stimulated their need to earn a wage through nursing; Wald, on the other hand, considered nursing as a life work after her rejection of admission to Vassar College. Yet each woman's written memoir, laced with hesitancy, portrays nursing as much more than a mere wage-earning endeavor. "Nursing work" was for them an opportunity to gain emotional satisfaction by understanding the kinship of mankind. Careful to tread between pure emotion and objective reason, they suggest a commitment to the *ideal* of nursing as paramount, while denying that nursing was an innate calling.[22]

Dock recalled that some years after sympathetically caring for her dying mother, she responded to a magazine clipping about Isabel Hampton Robb, as if drawn to a "familiar force of healing."[23] Goodrich remembered that she felt nursing to be a perfect outlet for her keen sense of responsibility and independence, even though "she hated sickness and had a horror of death."[24] Wald maintained that her exposure to a Bellevue graduate during her sister's pregnancy "awakened" her interest in nursing.[25]

The personal motivations of these women suggest that their choice of and commitment to nursing reflect a deeper sense of nursing than cognition alone would give. Subtly, their memoirs reveal that nursing provided them with an opportunity for a personal relationship with others, a way of encountering humanity in a face-to-face relationship, and a way of doing good works through the care of needy persons. Goodrich, with the most grandiloquent style of the three women, enthused that "the life of a nurse is indeed transfused with meaning who has by an iota furthered the end of those she serves."[26] More pragmatically, Wald wrote that "contact with ordinary people is a pleasurable satisfaction, for to keep the poor in your consciousness insures the power to transmit faith in a cause, to stir a response, and to change indifference."[27] Dock, expressing regrets, lamented that she lacked the "compassion and warm personal care" essential to good nursing.[28]

Although their transcendental idea of nursing can easily be dismissed as romantic or submissive, too cavalier an attitude toward the nurse inventors' compassionate attitude may obscure understanding. Encountering the underworld of the poor stimulated the nurse inventors to respond with compassion to human pain and misery. Compassion, in turn, became an expected attitude as nurse inventors created nursing practice within the context of Henry Street Settlement House. Their compassionate practice of nursing also served to quell personal restlessness, to offer individual creativity, and to create a purpose and a personal sense of meaning to their lives. Ideal nursing practice was tied to the causes of humanity and to the needs of the collective, which were larger than the individual nurse. And nursing was a means of reaching the goal of an improved society. As Wald wrote, "the nurse makes her contribution to human welfare unified and harmonized with those powers which aim at care and prevention."[29] Nursing, as an ideal, would accept a commitment to social causes and to the development of mankind's mind, body, and spirit.

Nursing legend and nursing history promote the idea that the nineteenth-century nurse was an extension of the pure, obedient, submissive Victorian woman who, as historian Susan Reverby notes, had "an obligation to care."[30] This view suggests that nursing's altruism manifested itself as an obsession with the behavior, the character, and the "being" of the individual nurse, while the "doing" of nursing, it is argued, was rigidly dictated by nurse leaders. The long history of hospital nursing's protracted focus on both the "character of the nurse" and on technique, which historian Ellen Baer calls the "procedure manual of nursing," supports the argument that goodness resided in the nurse who compliantly followed the procedures set by her superiors.[31]

In direct opposition to this traditional distinction, however, Wald, Dock, and Goodrich seemed to be contouring the ideal nature or virtue of nursing *practice,* which required some balanced union and synthesis of being and doing in order to care for others.[32] For the nurse inventors, societal and patient needs, rather than ordained procedures, determined the practice of nursing; the "being" of nursing was a group achievement and a group identity rather than a characteristic of an individual nurse. Nursing *practice* was not, according to Wald, Dock, and Goodrich, synonymous with "doing." Technical training was simply a component of the greater "nursing work," which concerned itself with human beings, relationships, and environment.[33] A bedbath was not a practice, but nursing was.[34] And the "being" of nursing belonged not to the individual nurse, but to the collective group called Nursing. This group identity, which Wald called the "spirit of nursing," was a virtue of nursing that enabled the profession, as a collective, to achieve the needed outcomes of nursing practice. The ideal outcome was conceptualized as a perfected humanity.

Prophetically, Wald feared the loss of the spirit of nursing. In 1908, fifteen years after the establishment of Henry Street Settlement House, Wald, confronted with Metropolitan Life Insurance Company's technocratic focus on money and efficient outcomes, lamented that "the lovely spirit of nursing" might be eroded if nursing colluded with the marketing scams of business.[35] Wald seemed to feel that the high ideals of improving humanity and the reality of bureaucracy would be at odds.

While the nurse inventors subscribed to the spirit of nursing as a virtue, they denied nursing *qua* religion. Goodrich's biographer, Harriet Koch, says that the elder Goodrich wanted her daughter to apply to St. Luke's Hospital (New York), but Annie proudly rebelled stating, "I will not go to a place where they ask if you belong to the Church."[36] And while careful to point out that she was raised in the Episcopal Church, Dock was equally vociferous in her rejection of religion and her acceptance of social justice:

> When I began to reflect, I saw that I had always had certain inarticulate instincts that were sound: a strong sympathy for the oppressed classes, a lively sense of justice, and a keen love of what we mean by freedom and liberty. . . . I had no religious beliefs and I felt no need of them. . . . The flash went through my mind: "there is not a good God." Instantly all regard for and belief in the Church as an institution fell from my mind as stone sinks in water, and never came back.[37]

Dock maintained that the old nursing sisters of the religious order, "closely confined in shackles of mental subjugation and social renunciation," held no hopes of creating a social order, but rather "gave their lives to an unquestioning service of devotion."[38] The key phrase for the nurse inventors was "unquestioning." Proponents of "purposeful and rational obedience" for worker nurses, Dock, Wald, and Goodrich shared an antipathy toward the authority of the church, while admiring, even finding solice within, "religious sentiment."[39] To these nurse inventors, the church's requirement of blind obedience negated emancipation for womanhood, diminished the hope of a better life for humans, and threatened Wald's ideal of nursing having a voice of its own.[40] Yet their zeal, bordering on dogmatic reverence, toward the attributes of compassion, respect, care, devotion, loyalty, harmony, essential dignity, and love seemed to accord them a commitment to some transcendent "other," to give them a feeling of personal importance and interiority, and to reveal to them the essential questions of human destiny. They created a conceptual boundary between secular and religious nursing and sought to justify its existence. Dock noted that:

> We belong to an age which is learning . . . the thrill of discovery that the human race is capable of improvement; that human society can be voluntarily and consciously built into a nobler and fairer form than those of the past. If now we have secured the freedom which was denied to the sister of the religious orders, we shirk its responsibilities and ignore its duties, but deliberately clothe ourselves again in her narrow-mindedness but without her holy zeal and self-consecration.[41]

The spirit of nursing, to the nurse inventors, was not the spark of organized religion, nor martyrdom, but a compassionate commitment to the human condition and to the rectification of the beautiful garbage of daily life. Iconoclastic at their core, the nurse inventors used the argument of nursing's social value as a battleground for their own doubts about wealth as a sign of worth, the meaning of human suffering, and their relationship with nature and the universe. In what seems to be an unveiling of her own wonderment with the nurse's role, Wald relayed a story of an ignorant, poor, suffering immigrant woman who was bewildered with the procedures of visiting a maternity center. Wald commented that the role of the nurse "can be perplexing to these women," but noted, with great relief and bemusement, that she knew an understanding had been gained when the immigrant woman commented, "I know what they are—sisters without religion."[42]

While religious sisters rejected the world and committed themselves to the spirit of God through caring, the nurse inventors, with secular superiority, rejected formal religion and committed themselves to reforming the world through the spirit of nursing. While the two sects approached their task from different perspectives, both nurses and sisters adopted a volitional attitude, dedicating themselves to the relief of others' pain. Yet to relieve pain, one must be drawn into it, to see it, to touch it, and to experience it. Nurses and sisters alike could not relieve pain through the safety of sentiment, but had to descend *into* the patients' lives so as to encounter the primal awesomeness of the human condition. Raw exposure to the beauty and the tragedy of lives promoted the hope that something—God and belief, or nursing and reform—gave life meaning. Thus, despite the nurse inventors' crafted conceptual boundaries to reject the religious nature of nursing, the irony is that both paths led all the sisters, nuns, and nurses alike deeper into the suffering world and, thereby, closer to a universal core that yearns to believe that life has meaning and purpose.

Belief and Unbelief

To rebuff religion, while espousing an exalting faith in civic humanism, progressivism, and the spirit of nursing, did not seem out of the ordinary for the nurse inventors. Before the middle of the nineteenth century, agnosticism and secularization in America seemed almost absurd, but soon unbelief emerged as an option within the general contours of society. According to James Turner, the urban landscape, coupled with advances in technology and science, disrupted society's relationship with nature and God.[43] While the clergy, by virtue of their office, traditionally served to explain the mysteries of life and reassure people about the unknowable, improved newspaper communication and increased travel allowed nineteenth-century Americans to choose points of view that differed from those of their village ministers and priests. Moreover, when universities such as Harvard replaced clerical presidents with professionals, the church's longstanding grip over education declined.

Although science and technology had begun to displace religion as an object of interest by the late 1860s, many "guardians of belief," particularly in the Northeast, sought to harmonize religion and science.[44] Advocates of using practical scientific knowledge to improve society, the moral guardians generated an avalanche of social reforms to reconcile human progress with divine sovereignty. And while "true" knowledge, that is, scientific knowledge, had to be verified by experience or experimentation, the idea that science complemented religion became popular. Science disclosed the laws of nature and being, and the discovery of a law presumed a lawgiver, namely God. Armed with such theories as Herbert Spencer's evolutionism and Auguste Comte's knowledge development, the idea that knowledge grows throughout history supported a belief of a supreme knower—a designer behind the design.[45] For a time it seemed possible that science and religion, bridged by reform, could cohabit and complement one another.

Yet, the conflict between science and religion was not resolved. Darwin's *Origin of the Species* applied an ax to even the strongest ties that bound science and religion. And while Darwin's treatise was published in 1859, the significance of the work, which historians continue to argue, affected the worldview for decades. Darwin showed how, through natural selection, organisms developed from the very simple to the extremely complex. The argument of design and, more important, the *Designer* of nature collapsed. Of course, it was still possible to believe in a god, but Darwin offered a plausible alternative explanation to the design theology. As Turner noted, without design, God did not vanish, but would have to be explained by faith rather than by reason and science.[46]

The raging arguments regarding Darwin and the relationship between science and religion threw some believers back to the source of knowledge that they knew—intuition. The believers argued that God remained impervious to human probing, and not even science could penetrate the essence of things that belonged to the Almighty. Still, as science principles became articulate and diffused into the culture, knowledge became associated with the practical, the touchable, and the measurable; God remained in the realm of belief and faith.[47]

By the Gilded Age, religion swelled with Gothic spires rising over American cities and church membership grew to new heights. Although doubters did not acquiesce to religion, they could not relinquish their grip on God without a replacement. Even for doubters, existence demanded some meaning and, thus, "morality" filled the void. Secularized morality, couched in the language of Leslie Stephen's *The Science of Ethics* (1882), argued that "we must love and serve one another."[48] Religious faith and intuition had nothing to do with morality, which, according to the doubters, was obviously based in reason and science. At the heart of this agnostic belief lay two principles—the nobility of the pursuit of truth and the commitment to human progress. As Turner says, progress did for unbelievers what faith did for believers.[49] One could feel that at death one's upright strivings did not evaporate into nothingness but had some moral worth in helping humanity toward higher limits. Truth and meaning, born of faith in God or belief in progress, became sacred.

Virtue as Compassion or Ethics?

The nurse inventors, born and raised in a social context that praised the morality of service to *Truth* (versus *t*ruths), human need, and progress, embraced those ideas from society that made them feel confident in transforming themselves and others. While denying the religious nature of nursing, they selected ideas from the social context that created sense of their lived experience. For Lillian Wald, the reality of life was an immersion in connectedness with the poor immigrants of New York's lower East Side. Remembering the window of opportunity that Henry Street Settlement House had given her life, she wrote years later:

> The East side called up a vague alarming picture of something strange and alien, a vast crowded area, a foreign city within our own for whose conditions we had no concern. Like the rest of the world, I had known little of it. . . . Past odorous fish stands, unregulated, uncovered garbage, and where children played lending themselves inevitably to all forms of inducing. All the maladjustments of our social and economic relations seemed epitomized in this brief journey.[50]

Assaulted by the lack of essential dignity of the conditions, but awestruck by the interdependence of mankind, she decided to bridge the gap. Living briefly at the College Settlement on Rivington Street, then at the top floor of a flat on Jefferson Street, and finally at the house at Henry Street, Wald and her colleagues lived and worked with the poor for nearly four decades. Outside established hospitals, "free from every form of control, without the benefit of managers, committees, medical encouragement, or police approval, there to do what we could do, to see what we could see, and to publicize all that was wrong and remediable by making the findings known," Wald professed herself a practical idealist who fashioned the spirit of nursing from ideas of "fellowship, harmony, and helping each other to the highest level."[51]

The virtues of what Wald hoped nursing to embody—morality, service, integrity, kinship of mankind, justice, and the art of humanity—

effectively denied religion while promoting a differentiated connectedness, a basic oneness, with humankind. The settlement house milieu fostered such a connection. As Dock observed, "Henry Street was perhaps like the pleasantest type of family life—a family to be sure, composed only of women, each one absorbed in busy interests, but in no sense . . . an institution."[52] Each nurse managed patients according "to her best judgment," and nursing practice problems were settled during evening conversation and consultation, "free of any kind of restrictive regulation."[53]

The spirit of nursing for Wald seemed to be akin to the Hebrew notion of *zedakah,* which literally means righteousness, but which usually is translated as compassion.[54] Compassion was not sentiment, but making justice and doing works of mercy. Compassion was not a favor to the poor, but something to which patients had a right, and for the nurse, an opportunity. Compassion was not pity, but celebration of the kinship of the human spirit. Compassion was not private, but public service. Compassion was not simply knowing about the suffering of others, but entering into it, sharing it, and understanding it. Compassion was not anti-intellectual, but sought to know and to understand the interconnections of all things. Compassion was not a commandment, but a spirituality that treated all creation with respect. Compassion was not an organized religion, but it was, for the nurse inventors, a way of life.[55]

Historian Susan Reverby noted that nursing lacked a "conception of nursing as an occupational sisterhood built on caring and the demand for rights" and instead adopted the "need to accept obligations, duties," and thus, exploitation.[56] Yet, this particular thought collective, connected with Henry Street Settlement House, had a vision of nursing as a sisterhood with a core value of compassionate care of humanity *without* the self-sacrifice demanded by organized religion. The terms humanity, progress, fellowship, civic righteousness, unfailing goodness, and ethics—language distinctive of the era—supported the view that the "spirit of nursing" was compassion.

Writing in 1900, Dock noted that she had once advocated establishing a code of ethics as one of the first duties for organizing an association of nurses, but after consideration she withdrew that claim.[57] With a newfound insight that a codified set of ethics was restrictive, Dock proposed that if nurses lived in an ethical manner, consistent with the norms of nursing practice, they would not need a code. Ethical life was more than maxims, just as an intellectual life was more than booklearning. Moreover, Dock, referring to expected nurse behavior within hospitals, indignantly maintained that ethics encompassed more than etiquette. An ethical life was a comprehensive approach to human beings. "If nurses walked in the spirit of truth and justice principles, the slavishness of obedience and moral cowardice of subordination would be unnecessary."[58] Dock, using the terms *truth* and *justice*, urged that nurses become internally motivated and identify with nursing's commitment to compassion rather than follow a set of rules called ethics. She maintained that obedience for either the sake of obedience or for a worthless cause deteriorated character, "preventing initiative, independent thought, and self-reliant action."[59] Only when obedience became a symbol of an understanding that all humans were connected and that "the slave stands on the level with himself" could a nurse make a contribution to the goal of unified human welfare.[60]

Echoing Dock's beliefs, Goodrich argued that the ethical significance of nursing "is indeed its vitalizing force," so much so that "it is consistent to assert that the terms *good* and *ethical* as applied to nursing practice are synonymous."[61] The nurse, according to the dramatic Goodrich, "stood at the gateway of life and death," and it was this critical position that demanded "the fullest understanding of all that pertains to the creative task to which she has aspired."[62] Goodrich also denounced etiquette as a synonym of ethics, pointing out that producing a better world, rather than politeness, was life's overall ethical objective. The nurse, as an interpreter of life, ministered to the sick, and these acts of compassion verified that "the calling, vocation, profession, what you will, is in itself intrinsically ethical."[63] Nursing, as an exemplification of compassion toward human suffering, hoped to "heal the body with perchance to save the soul."[64]

The three nurse inventors, exposed to life, death, and the tragedies of human existence on the New York City streets, could neither tranquilize themselves with the trivial nor live wholly in the dimension of the visible. Like many humans, they sought meaning in their lives. Hoping to transcend human vulnerability and yearning to be part of a greater and higher whole, they did not search upward to heaven and organized religion, but embraced earthly ideas of reform, compassion, and progress as a means to redeem humanity—and to construct nursing. Yet all true religions embrace the words *humanity* and *compassion* as an expression of the commitment to a transcendent other who integrates one's life. Thus, both nursing and religion, if pursued compassionately, healed wounded minds, bodies, and spirits. Although the nurse inventors intended an unyielding boundary between religion and nursing, the kindred missions of religion and nursing rendered the boundary translucent.

Conclusions

Early in the twentieth century a thought collective of nursing espoused the idea that compassion toward humanity was the core value within nursing. While they denied nursing as a manifestation of conventional religion, Dock, Wald, and Goodrich promoted the notion that compassion was a necessary condition to the "being" of a nurse. They envisioned that secular nursing would emulate the values of the religious sisters without accepting their rules, regulations, and cloistered life. Compassion, once associated with God's authority, would, according to the nurse inventors, be replaced with compassion based on commitment to the authority of humanity and its social progress.

As in most historical research, this is not the end of the story, but rather the beginning. While the idea of compassion as a nursing virtue can be identified within the thought collective of Dock, Wald, and Goodrich, there is plentiful evidence that diversity of thinking among nurses exists through time. Other leaders, such as Harriet Lounsbery (1899), Isabel Hampton Robb (1900), S. Lillian Clayton (1916), and Eva Allerton (1898), writing on the topic of ethics, suggest that the intimacy inherent in nursing practice required religious goodness, trust, the idea of discipline, and obedience. Confronted with the reality of pupil nurses who did not demonstrate the necessary goodness, compassion metamorphosed into ethics, which, in turn, became a set of "rules" of conduct. With these shifts in thinking, the conceptual boundaries between compassion and ethics, between behavior and character, between being a nurse and acting like a nurse, between spiritual development and compliance, between excellence and submission, between commitment to mankind and veneration of leaders, between individuality and perfection, and between teaching and controlling became diffuse and riddled with angst.[65] As Susan Reverby observed, the "theoretical and moral power of nursing," which this article argues was compassion, became devalued and mutated, reduced to a rather rigid rule orientation of nurse leaders.[66] Compassion became compulsion.

And while Reverby analyzes how this "character as ideology" emerged, nurses want to believe that compassion, as a core of nursing, lay dormant (or not so dormant) throughout the decades. The history of nurses' diverse thinking patterns, as well as the social, economic, political, and intellectual factors that influenced changes in thought, is yet to be written. As the century draws to a close, nurses are seeking to reexamine, reframe, and clarify the heritage and tradition of nursing. And once again, the idea of compassion and caring as a central virtue in nursing appeals to the core of nurses. The traditional tenet that "nursing was born in the church . . ." may well be a truism. Or as Matthew Fox notes, "you may call God love, you may call God goodness, but God is best described as compassion."[67]

DIANE HAMILTON, PhD, RN
School of Nursing
University of Rochester
601 Elmwood Avenue Box HWH
Rochester, N.Y. 14642
Phone: (716) 275-8876

Acknowledgments

Grateful acknowledgment is made to Lillian Brunner and Joan Lynaugh for their significant contributions to this study. The research was supported by The Lillian Sholtis Brunner Summer Fellowship for Historical Research in Nursing offered by the Center for the Study of the History of Nursing at the University of Pennsylvania.

Notes

1. Teresa Christy, *Cornerstone for Nursing Education: A History of the Division of Nursing Education of Teachers College, Columbia University, 1899–1947* (New York: Teachers College Press, 1969); Joanne Ashley, *Hospitals, Paternalism and the Role of the Nurse* (New York: Teachers College Press, 1976); Janet Mottus, *New York Nightingales: The Emergence of the Nursing Profession at Bellevue and New York Hospital, 1850–1920* (Ann Arbor, Mich.: UMI Research Press, 1981); Barbara Melosh, *The Physicians' Hand: Work, Culture, and Conflict in American Nursing* (Philadelphia: Temple University Press, 1982); Patricia O'Brien, "All a Woman's Life Can Bring: the Domestic Roots of Nursing In Philadelphia," *Nursing Research* 36, no. 1 (January/February 1987): 12–17; Susan Reverby, *Ordered to Care: The Dilemma of American Nursing, 1850–1945* (Cambridge, Mass.: Cambridge University Press, 1987); Charles Rosenberg, *The Care of Strangers: The Rise of America's Hospital System* (New York: Basic Books, 1987); Joan Lynaugh and Claire Fagin, "Coming of Age or Coming Apart: Nursing in the 20th Century," *Image* 20, no. 4, (Winter 1988): 184–88.

2. H. S. Kim, *The Nature of Theoretical Thinking in Nursing* (Norwalk, Conn.: Appleton-Century-Crofts, 1983), 9; Afaf Meleis, *Theoretical Nursing: Development and Progress* (Philadelphia, Pa.: J. B. Lippincott, 1985), 37.

3. U.S. Department of Commerce, Bureau of Census, *Historical Statistics of*

the United States: Colonial Times to 1957 (Washington, D.C., 1960), 34; Lavinia Dock and Isabel Stewart, *A Short History of Nursing* (New York: G. P. Putnam's Sons, 1920), 162–66.

4. The history of the concept and emergence of professions is well documented. See Robert Wiebe, *The Search for Order, 1877–1920* (New York: Hill and Wang, 1967); Magali Sarfatti Larson, *The Rise of Professionalism: A Sociological Analysis* (Berkeley: University of California Press, 1977); Roy Lubove, *The Professional Altruist: The Emergence of Social Work as a Career, 1880–1930* (New York: Atheneum, 1972); Alexander Oleson and John Voss, eds., *The Organization of Knowledge in Modern America* (Baltimore, Md.: The Johns Hopkins University Press, 1979); Thomas Haskell, *The Emergence of Professional Social Science: The American Social Science Association and the Nineteenth-Century Crises of Authority* (Urbana: University of Illinois Press, 1977); Burton Bledstein, *The Culture of Professionalism: The Middle Class and the Development of Higher Education in America* (New York: W. W. Norton and Co., 1979).

5. Ian Hacking, *Reconstructing Individualism* (Stanford, Calif.: Stanford University Press, 1985).

6. Ludwig Fleck, *The Genesis and Development of a Scientific Fact* (Chicago: University of Chicago Press, 1979), 25, 38–51.

7. The literature of the sociology of knowledge is a large body of work. For a beginning discussion, See Emile Durkheim, *De la Divisíon du Travail Social: Etude sur l'Organisation des Sociétés Superiéures,* translated by George Simpson (Paris: Alcan, 1893) [Translation, 1933]; Fleck, *Genesis and Development of a Scientific Fact;* Thomas Kuhn, *The Structure of Scientific Revolutions* (Chicago: University of Chicago Press, 1962); Mary Douglas, *Implicit Meanings* (London: Routledge and Kegan Paul, 1975); Mary Douglas, *How Institutions Think* (Syracuse, N.Y.: Syracuse University Press, 1986).

8. It is beyond not only the scope but the ability of the author to solve the problem of dualistic thinking. Currently, it is a topic of many articles, seminars, conferences, and think tanks within many disciplines. For a discussion of the dilemma as it relates to history of ideas, see John Toews, "Intellectual History after the Linguistic Turn," *American Historical Review* 92, no. 4 (October 1987): 879–907; Eric Fuhrman, *A Sociology of Knowledge in America, 1883–1915* (Charlottesville: University of Virginia Press, 1980); David Hollinger, *In the American Province* (Baltimore, Md.: The Johns Hopkins University Press, 1985); Dominick LaCapra, *Rethinking Intellectual History: Text, Contexts, Language* (Ithaca, N.Y.: Cornell University Press, 1983); Henrika Kuklick, "The Sociology of Knowledge: Retrospect and Prospect," *Annals Reviews of Sociology* 9 (1983): 287–310.

9. LaCapra, *Rethinking Intellectual History,* 36.

10. Christy, *Cornerstone for Nursing Education,* 3–29.

11. Henry Commager, *The American Mind* (New Haven, Conn.: Yale University, 1952), 212.

12. Wiebe, *Search for Order,* 3–21.

13. Jane Addams, *Twenty Years at Hull House* (New York: Macmillan Co., 1938), 90–101.

14. Public health has a rich history of its own. The orientation of public health

has experienced changes, which to some authors is a commentary on social, political, economic, and intellectual shifts within the American social system. See Allen Davis, *Spearheads of Reform: The Social Settlements and the Progressive Movement, 1890–1914* (New York: Oxford University Press, 1967); Barbara Rosencrantz, *Public Health and the State: Changing Views in Massachusetts, 1842–1936* (Cambridge, Mass.: Harvard University Press, 1972); John Duffy, *A History of Public Health in New York City, 1866–1966* (New York: Russell Sage Foundation, 1974); George Rosen, *Preventive Medicine in the United States: 1900–1975* (New York: Prodist, 1977); Karen Buhler-Wilkerson, *False Dawn: The Rise and Decline of Public Health Nursing, 1900–1930* (PhD diss., University of Pennsylvania, 1984).

15. William O'Neill, *Everyone Was Brave: A History of Feminism in America* (New York: Quandrangle, 1971), 77–106; Ellen Condliffe Lagemann, *A Generation of Women: Social Feminism in the 1920's* (Cambridge, Mass.: Harvard University Press), 154–59; Barbara Welter, "The Cult of True Womanhood: 1800–1860," *American Quarterly* 18 (Summer 1966); Caroll Smith-Rosenberg, *Disorderly Conduct: Visions of Gender in Victorian America* (New York: Oxford University Press, 1985), 77–89, 167–77; Susan Armeny, "Organized Nurses, Women Philanthropists, and the Intellectual Bases for Cooperation Among Women, 1898–1920," in *The New Nursing History,* ed. Ellen Lagemann (New York: Teachers College, Columbia University, 1983), 13–35.

16. For an overview of nurses who contributed to nursing between the years 1890–1900, see Vern Bullough, Olga Church, and Alice Stein, *American Nursing: A Biographical Dictionary,* vol. 1 (New York: Garland Publishing, 1988) and Vern Bullough, Lilli Sentz, and Alice Stein, *America Nursing: A Biographical Dictionary,* vol. 2 (New York: Garland Press, 1992).

17. Fleck, *Genesis of a Scientific Fact,* 192.

18. Lavinia Dock, "Some Urgent Social Claims," *American Journal of Nursing* 1 (January 1907): 895–905.

19. Annie Goodrich, "The Nurse and the University," *The Social and Ethical Significance of Nursing* (New York: MacMillan, 1932), 334.

20. Lillian Wald, *Windows on Henry Street* (Boston, Mass.: Little and Brown, 1934), 75–78.

21. Although Mary Roberts, longtime editor of the *American Journal of Nursing,* called Goodrich, Wald, and M. Adelaide Nutting the "Triumvirate," the Henry Street tie, which eluded Nutting, may be important in terms of how a certain set of nursing ideas formed. Moreover, Dock, Goodrich, and Wald did produce a collection of ideas in book form. While Nutting published articles and certainly wrote two chapters of Nutting and Dock's classic history, *A History of Nursing,* Dock's ideas predominate in both the four volume and the short version of her treatise. In addition to Dock's two works, Goodrich's classic, *Social and Ethical Significance of Nursing,* and Wald's two works on Henry Street Settlement House, *House on Henry Street* and *Windows on Henry Street,* form a grouping of nursing "texts" that are a reasonable starting point for ideas on history of nursing. Of course, the choice of Wald, Dock, and Goodrich as a thought collective is not sacrosanct. Dock and Stewart, *A Short History of Nursing;* Lavinia Dock and M. Adelaide Nutting, *A History of Nursing,* vols. 1–4 (New York: Putnam, 1912); Annie Goodrich, *The Social*

and Ethical Significance of Nursing (New York: MacMillan, 1932); Lillian Wald, *House on Henry Street* (New York: Henry Holt and Co., 1915); Wald, *Windows on Henry Street*.

22. Ibid.

23. Lavinia Dock, "Lavinia L. Dock: Self-Portrait," *Nursing Outlook* 25 (January 1977): 23–26.

24. Harriet Berger Koch, *Militant Angel* (New York: MacMillan, 1951) 14.

25. Wald, *House on Henry Street,* 12–16.

26. Goodrich, *Social and Ethical Significance of Nursing,* 10.

27. Wald, *House on Henry Street,* 10.

28. Dock, "Lavinia L. Dock: Self-Portrait," 24.

29. Wald, *House on Henry Street,* 60.

30. Nurse historians, for the most part, cite this argument. See Reverby, *Ordered to Care*.

31. Dr. Ellen D. Baer, telephone conversation with author, 10 February 1992.

32. The term nursing practice was called "nursing work" by the nurse inventors. Anne Bishop and John Scuder, *The Practical, Moral, and Personal Sense of Nursing: A Phenomenological Philosophy of Practice* (Albany, N.Y.: State University Press, 1990), 173.

33. The nurse inventors were clear that the mechanics of nursing and the profession of nursing were distinctly different. Goodrich, quoting public health Professor C. E. A. Winslow, liked to say that a nurse must not be "simply an empirically trained upper bedside servant, but understand the 'laws and principles' of science." See Goodrich, *The Social and Ethical Significance of Nursing,* 34. They believed that every nurse needed a broad education so as to grasp the responsibility of their life work: namely, moving the human race toward essential dignity, health, and well-being. Dock used the dualistic language "technical training versus theoretical teaching, nursing versus routine hospital work, details of work versus the spirit of nursing." See Lavinia Dock, "Nursing Organization in Germany and England," "The Nurses' Settlement in New York," and "Ethics or a Code of Ethics?" *Short Papers On Nursing Subjects,* in *A Lavinia Dock Reader,* ed. Janet James (1900; reprint, New York: Garland Press, 1985), 16–26, 27–30, 37–40. Also, see Lavinia Dock, "Hospital Organization," *National Hospital Record* 6 (1903): 10–14. In Goodrich's language, "the complete nurse implied attainments in special knowledge as distinguished from mere skill. To effectively interpret life, neither a liberal education nor a high degree of technical skill will suffice. She must be a master of two tongues: of science and of the people." See Goodrich, *The Social and Ethical Significance of Nursing,* 14, 38, 70. And Wald was also clear that the service of the nurse's mind, heart, and hands led to the social betterment of mankind. See: Wald, *House on Henry Street,* 336.

34. Alasdair MacIntyre, *After Virtue* (Notre Dame, Ind.: University of Notre Dame Press, 1984), 187; Bishop and Scuder, *Practical, Moral, and Personal Sense of Nursing,* 13–28.

35. Diane Hamilton, "Cost of Caring," *Bulletin of the History of Medicine* 63 (Spring 1989): 414–34.

36. Koch, *Militant Angel,* 14.

37. Dock, "Lavinia L. Dock: Self-Portrait," 15.

38. Dock, "Some Urgent Social Claims," 895–905.

39. Dock, "Ethics or a Code of Ethics?," 56–57; Mary Roberts, "Lavinia Lloyd Dock, Nurse, Feminist, Internationalist," *American Journal of Nursing* 56 (February 1956): 176–79; Goodrich, *Social and Ethical Significance of Nursing,* 8–9; Wald, *House on Henry Street,* 117.

40. Wald, *Windows on Henry Street,* 75.

41. Roberts, "Lavinia Lloyd Dock, Nurse, Feminist, Internationalist," 176–79.

42. Wald, *Windows on Henry Street,* 92–95.

43. James Turner, *Without God, Without Creed: The Origins of Unbelief in America* (Baltimore, Md.: The Johns Hopkins University Press, 1985), 116.

44. Turner, *Without God, Without Creed,* 124.

45. Lavinia Dock was a reader, if not admirer, of Herbert Spencer, as was Annie Goodrich, who also had a particular fondness for Tolstoy. For a discussion of the whole controversy, which included Spencer, Darwin, and Aggisiz, see Turner, *Without God, Without Creed,* 150–72; John Hedley Brooke, *Science and Religion* (New York: Cambridge University Press, 1991).

46. The arguments regarding Darwin and the relationship between science and religion are numerous and varied. See Richard Hofstader, *Social Darwinism in American Thought* (Boston, Mass.: Boston University, 1955); Charles Rosenberg, *No Other Gods: On Science and American Social Thought* (Baltimore, Md.: The Johns Hopkins University Press, 1976); Herbert Hovenkamp, *Science and Religion in America: 1800–1860* (Philadelphia: University of Pennsylvania Press, 1978); Bernard Lightman, *The Origins Of Agnosticism, Victorian Unbelief, and the Limits of Knowledge* (Baltimore, Md.: The Johns Hopkins University Press, 1978); John Cerello, *The Secularization of the Soul* (Philadelphia: University of Pennsylvania Press, 1982); Brooke, *Science and Religion.*

47. Turner, *Without God, Without Creed,* 202.

48. Leslie Stephen, *The Science of Ethics* (New York: MacMillan, 1882), 32–36.

49. Turner, *Without God, Without Creed,* 217–20.

50. Wald, *Windows on Henry Street,* 3–6.

51. Lillian Wald to unknown person, 31 May 1922, Welfare Division Files, Metropolitan Life Insurance Company Archives, New York City; Wald, *Windows on Henry Street,* 118.

52. Dock, "The Nurses' Settlement in New York," 27–36.

53. Ibid.

54. William Eckhardt, *Compassion: Toward a Science of Value* (Toronto: CPRI Press, 1973), 258.

55. Matthew Fox, *A Spirituality Named Compassion* (San Francisco, Calif.: Harper, 1979).

56. Susan Reverby notes that character as skill became the ideology of the nursing discipline and argues that if the conception of nursing had been based on rights and caring rather than obligation and duty, nursing would have had the ideological material necessary to guard against exploitation. I am arguing that within this particular thought collective the idea of caring and compassion was indeed the ideological base, but do agree with Reverby that it slowly (or not so

slowly) mutated, maybe within the contexts of institutional bureaucracy, to become compliance or an "obligation to care." See Reverby, *Ordered to Care,* 58.

57. Dock, "Ethics or a Code of Ethics?" 37–57.

58. Ibid.

59. Ibid.

60. Ibid.

61. Goodrich, *The Social and Ethical Significance of Nursing,* 3–5.

62. Ibid.

63. Ibid., 1–15.

64. Ibid.

65. For a very nice collection of nurse authorship on the topic of ethics, see Nettie Birnbach and Sandra Lewenson, eds., *First Words: Selected Addresses from the National League for Nursing, 1894–1933* (New York: National League for Nursing, 1992), 197–234. Also see Isabel Hampton Robb, *Nursing Ethics For Hospital and Private Use* (Cleveland, Ohio: E. C. Koeckert, 1990), and Harriet Lounsbery, *Nursing Ethics* (New York: Appleton, 1889).

66. Reverby, *Ordered to Care,* 58–59.

67. Fox, *A Spirituality Named Compassion,* 34.

White Nurses, Black Midwives, and Public Health in Mississippi, 1920–1950

Susan L. Smith
Department of History
University of Alberta

Introduction

Black lay midwives were important health workers well beyond their midwifery role in southern rural areas in the first half of the twentieth century. They were part of a black community health network, including ministers, teachers, and a few black nurses and doctors, that provided health education and health services to African-Americans. Lay midwives worked primarily with women and children, the key targets of public health work, and they also provided health education to the entire community. Midwives proved to be a vital link between poor African-Americans and health departments. Indeed, the success of official state and county health projects among African-Americans depended on the work of black midwives.[1]

In the past few decades, the burgeoning interest among scholars in the study of lay midwives has deepened our understanding of the history of health care in the United States. Much of the literature has focused on native-born whites and European immigrants, although there is a growing body of material about African-American midwives.[2] This article examines the complex relationship between public health nurses and lay midwives in African-American communities in Mississippi from 1920 to 1950. Based on records of the Mississippi State Board of Health, including public health nurses' reports and correspondence from midwives, this essay places the activities of nurses and midwives at the center of the story of public health work. Nurses, most of whom were white, and midwives, most of whom were black, worked together to implement the modern public health care system in Mississippi and other southern states.

Ironically, state regulation of midwifery, which brought public health

Nursing History Review 2 (1994): 29–49.

nurses in close contact with lay midwives, led to the creation of an unexpected cadre of public health workers for the state. Beginning in the 1920s, Mississippi enacted state restrictions on midwifery practice as health officials identified midwives as a public health problem. Public health officials claimed that midwives did not maintain clean environments and that they used unscientific, and therefore unsafe, folk medicine. Yet, health officers and public health nurses soon discovered that midwives provided valuable assistance in implementing health policy in black communities. Even though nurses never treated midwives as their equals, they did frequently note midwife contributions to public health work.[3]

Examining the health work of midwives demonstrates the significant contributions made by poor black women to the implementation of state health programs. Midwives assisted nurses with health education, promotion of clinics and immunization programs, and efforts to encourage women to receive prenatal and postnatal medical examinations. Midwives and public health nurses developed a reciprocal relationship in which midwives aided the work of nurses, even as nurses provided them with training. Health reform in Mississippi, therefore, developed out of a dynamic relationship between public health professionals, midwives, and clients.[4]

The Midwives of Mississippi

Across the nation, lay midwives delivered half of all babies as late as 1910. Much of their practice was among European immigrant women and southern black women. By 1930, with immigration restrictions and the preference of urban women for childbirth attendance by physicians, midwives delivered only 15 percent of all births.[5] At that time, 80 percent of all remaining midwives practiced in the South, where midwives delivered over one-fourth of all babies and over one-half of black babies. Even as midwifery declined in significance in northeastern and midwestern urban areas, the number of practicing midwives did not drop significantly in the South until after 1950.[6]

In Mississippi, where half the population was black, the vast majority of midwives were black women. Black midwives, called "granny" midwives by white health officials, delivered most of the black babies and even a few of the white babies in the state. In Mississippi in the late 1920s, midwives delivered 8 percent of white babies and 80 percent of black babies, and although they delivered only 5 percent of white babies by the 1940s, they continued to deliver 80 percent of black babies.[7]

Scholars have demonstrated the important role black midwives played in their communities in cultural transmission and community leadership, as well as in health care. Midwives were highly respected, prestigious members of the communities they served, even if they were at the bottom of the medical hierarchy. Midwives were the female counterparts to preachers as the most influential members of the community. They were at the center of traditional healing networks in rural black communities of the South, and served as advisers and spiritual leaders. Midwifery was only part of the labor they performed, for most midwives also cared for their own families, tended crops in the fields, and worked as domestic servants or teachers.[8]

Black women, and some white, preferred midwife over physician deliveries for economic and cultural reasons. Midwives were cheaper than doctors and would travel to remote places. Midwives provided comfort and support to pregnant women before, during, and after delivery. They even looked after the cooking and cleaning, in addition to caring for the mother and newborn. Many women preferred delivery by another woman, especially one with a reputation for skillful service. Finally, midwives treated birthing women among the rural poor with dignity rather than disregard.[9]

Because they believed that they did God's work, many midwives did not insist on payment, although a few dollars or payment in kind, such as a gift of pigs, was typical. One woman in Alabama gave her cow to the midwife for her delivery because her husband could not pay the fee.[10] In the 1920s, midwife Bessie Sutton received about $1.50 for a delivery, and when she retired in 1962 the fee had increased to $20. She explained that she did not do the work for the money but because she loved people. She emphasized, "If I'd a stopped 'cause they didn't pay me, I'd a stopped a long time ago."[11]

Midwife Training Campaigns and Public Health Nurses

Midwives and public health nurses together implemented the development of a modern public health care system in Mississippi. As midwives came under state regulation beginning in the early 1920s they developed a working relationship with public health nurses who were responsible for midwife training campaigns to "modernize" midwifery. Intervention of the state into the previously unregulated practice of midwifery meant the creation of a division between state-sanctioned midwives and those midwives identified by the state as unfit to practice and therefore vulnerable to prosecution, such as uncooperative women and any men. Whether or not midwives abided by the new regulations, the state placed limitations on the health services midwives were entitled to perform during childbirth and in general.

In 1921 Laurie Jean Reid, a white nurse with the United States Public Health Service (USPHS), came to Mississippi to survey the midwives of the state. Reid traveled around the eighty-two counties of Mississippi tracking down the names of midwives and registering the women county by county. She identified over 4,000 midwives in Mississippi, and the state located an additional 1,000 midwives a few years later.[12] As she explained to the white Mississippi State Medical Association, her purpose was to address the fact that the United States had higher infant and maternal mortality rates than many European countries. Reid advised that these rates were caused by poor health care for pregnant women from "careless physicians and by illiterate and ignorant midwives."[13] Sidestepping the issue of physician care, she proposed that the state eliminate those midwives who were too old to be educated, and register and train those who remained. Targeting midwives was an easier solution for public health officials dealing with an impoverished rural population than criticizing physician care or altering the economic and living conditions that contributed to ill-health.[14]

Despite the fact that health officials blamed midwives for maternal and infant deaths, their safety record was not any worse than that of physicians. Some contemporary studies even showed that maternal mortality rates were lowest where the percentage of midwife-attended births was highest.[15] In 1923 Nurse Supervisor Lois Trabert of Mississippi's Bureau of Child Hygiene proclaimed: "I firmly believe that when we do get these midwives properly trained, in as far as that is possible, that they will do better and cleaner work than the average country doctor."[16] By the 1930s, the Mississippi Board of Health employed 125 white public health nurses and 6 black public health nurses to train lay midwives.[17]

From 1910 to 1930, health reformers and medical professionals engaged in a debate over the future of midwives, with some obstetricians arguing for their immediate elimination and public health officials arguing that midwives were needed, even if only temporarily.[18] Most public health doctors and nurses in Mississippi supported the gradual, not immediate, elimination of midwives, believing that they were a "necessary evil" until there were enough hospitals and doctors to care for rural women.

The decision to regulate, and only rarely eliminate, lay midwives rested on the fact that southern, rural areas had an inadequate number of practicing physicians to serve as the sole childbirth attendants. Midwives were available where physicians were not. Between 1920 and 1950, there were consistently twice as many midwives as physicians in Mississippi, with at least 2,000 to 4,000 black and several hundred white registered midwives, and only 1,000 to 1,800 practicing physicians, less than 75 of whom were black.[19] Other southern states reported equal or greater numbers of practicing midwives, including approximately 3,000 in Alabama, 4,000 to 9,000 in North Carolina, 5,000 to 6,000 in Georgia, and perhaps as many as 10,000 in Florida. All of these figures are rough estimates because health officials had no definite idea of the number of unregistered midwives who delivered babies.[20]

Southern state boards of health argued that training midwives lowered mortality rates. For example, Dr. Felix J. Underwood, the executive officer of the Mississippi State Board of Health from 1924 to 1958, pointed to the decline in state maternal and infant mortality rates. The total maternal mortality rates for the state dropped from 9.5 per 1,000 deliveries in 1921 to 4.4 in 1942, with black rates dropping from 12 in 1921 to 5.5 in 1942. A similar pattern held for infant mortality rates, which are the number of deaths per 1,000 live births in the first year of life. These rates dropped from 68 in 1921 to 47 in 1942 for the state as a whole, and from 85 to 54 for black infants in the corresponding years.[21]

Board of Health's Educational Programs

From 1920 to 1950, public health nurses implemented the board of health's educational programs, using midwife manuals that carried virtually the same message for three decades.[22] The lessons taught by the nurses emphasized limitations on midwives and the ultimate authority of doctors. Above all else, the two issues on which nurses focused were: (1) the importance of cleanliness, and (2) the need to call on a physician in case of complications during delivery. Before state training began, midwives wore whatever they chose and carried the tools of their trade in an assortment of bags, such as flour sacks. Nurses permitted midwives to continue carrying midwife bags, but they had to upgrade them from flour sacks to black leather bags. Nurses instructed the midwife to perform deliveries wearing a clean white dress, with a white mask and white paper cap, which nurses taught them to make to keep hair out of the way. The nurses also insisted that midwives keep their hands and nails clean.[23]

State boards of health in the North as well as the South followed a similar pattern of midwife instruction. Mississippi and other states required midwives to file birth certificates for each birth they attended, therefore requiring illiterate women to find someone else to fill out the forms. Nurses forbade midwives to use any folk medicine or herbal remedies in their childbirth work. In addition, in order to prevent infections nurses instructed midwives not to perform any digital examination of women during labor; only doctors were allowed to put their hands into the birth canal. If midwives followed this rule, they no doubt had difficulty identifying how much a woman's cervix had dilated and the progression of labor.

Some of the nurses' instructions conflicted with longstanding midwifery practices and therefore resulted in midwife resistance. For example, nurses insisted that midwives deliver women on the bed and not the floor. Mothers and midwives particularly resisted this requirement because many women felt the urge to walk around during labor and found it more comfortable to deliver in a squatting position, assisted by gravity. Furthermore, some midwives preferred to keep the bed clean and have all the mess on the floor. Alabama midwife Margaret Smith explained why she ignored the rule. As she pointed out, "when you in misery, if there is any way you can ease that misery, you gonna ease it."[24]

Nurses intended to ensure compliance with these rules by occasionally supervising deliveries and inspecting midwife bags. However, midwives were not always cooperative. Former county health officer Dr. W. E. Riecken, Jr., recalled that some midwives engaged in the practice of "a bag to show and a bag to go." Midwives used this strategy to circumvent the rules by keeping "a clean, properly organized bag for inspection and licensing and . . . another that was used for deliveries."[25] Nurse Elsie Davis mentioned in 1931 that some of the midwives with whom she worked refused to bring their bags for inspection, while others did not maintain their bags in sterile condition, offering the excuse that they just came off duty.[26] Nurses even inspected midwives' homes to see that they understood the principles of cleanliness. Nurses Abbie G. Hall and Caroline Bourg of Sharkey and Issaquena counties reported: "We try to always keep in mind our midwives and never miss an opportunity to stop at their homes and inspect bags whenever we are in the neighborhood."[27]

Midwives resented nurses' implications that they had not performed their work well before regulation by the state. As midwife Otha Bell Jones of Itta Bena explained in 1938, she had learned how to be a midwife twenty-three years earlier through apprenticing with midwife Nancy Wright. "And dear friends," she wrote the board of health, "I had nursed 36 womens before I got any permit and I has fill the sum of 15 books with 25 leaves each." Despite her long lists of women she had delivered, she wrote: "[I] never lose a woman in childbirth since I have started out."[28] Midwife Onnie Lee Logan attended her midwife training classes and received some instruction, but she emphasized that "two-thirds of what I know about deliverin', carin' for mother and baby, what to expect, what was happenin' and was goin' on, I didn't get it from the class. God gave it to me. So many things I got from my own plain motherwit."[29] Yet, another midwife observed that even though she had a great deal of experience, she could still learn more. "Each time I attend my monthly meeting I learn something new, and I am happy to admit that because so many won't."[30]

Midwife Monthly Club Meetings

Beginning in the 1920s, the state required midwives to have monthly club meetings at which they were to further their knowledge. Dressed in their white delivery outfits, the women were supposed to read from the state's midwife manual and discuss any delivery problems they encountered. Although public health nurses initially organized the local clubs, the meetings were run entirely by midwives. Each midwife club selected a leader or president and a secretary, and they were in charge of reporting the minutes of the meeting to the county public health nurse or, if there was none, to the state supervisor of midwives. The midwife leader ran inspection of the midwives' bags and fingernails and handed out silver nitrate eye drops to prevent blindness in newborns caused by passing through the birth canal of mothers with gonorrhea.[31]

Midwife meetings had definite religious overtones. Usually midwives held the meetings in churches, one of the few public buildings controlled by African-Americans in rural communities. For example, the midwives of Hub, Mississippi, met monthly at Sweet Valley Baptist Church.[32] Midwife leaders also ran the meetings like a church service, complete with opening prayer and song, a reading from the Bible, short readings from "the Book," or midwife manual, and singing of the midwife songs. Midwife songs included "Protect the Mother and Baby," sung to the tune of "Mary Had A Little Lamb," which had hand motions to go along with the lyrics describing the importance of clean clothes, clean hands, clean midwives.[33] In 1937

John Lomax, a native of Holmes County and curator of folk songs at the Library of Congress, recorded a dozen midwives singing such songs at the Mississippi State Board of Health.[34]

Even though midwives seemed to have enjoyed the opportunity to socialize with each other, share stories, and sing together, they could not always attend every monthly meeting. Attendance was always down during times of heavy field labor and when weather made travel difficult, especially for women who had to walk several miles to the meetings. In 1923 Nurse Agnes B. Belser reported: "I have had but one midwife meeting as they begged off because of the cotton picking season."[35] Another nurse, Louise James, mentioned that her "greatest trouble in having a full attendance was caused by this season being cane grinding season and most all old women are used to skim cane syrup. Very often I had to go to the mill to get my entire class."[36] Despite the difficulty maintaining attendance, the number of midwife clubs increased over the years, growing from 290 clubs in the state in 1928 to 505 in 1942.[37]

Registration for Permits and Regulation of Midwife Practice

Midwives were careful about state rules regarding registration for permits and regulation of midwife practice. They took the issue of registration very seriously, identifying themselves in correspondence by their permit numbers, as requested by the state. Midwives were cautious because the state threatened to revoke the permits of women who did not follow the regulations. In 1923 Mississippi Nurse Mae Reeves indicated that some nurses "found one midwife treating gynecological cases and children. We revoked her permit."[38] In 1924 a nurse in Washington County reported: "In follow up work for midwives found that one had delivered case without cap and gown, and had also made [digital] examination. Her permit was revoked for one month and at the end of that month she is not to take a case unless I can be with her at time of delivery."[39] Punishment for performing digital exams and failing to wear regulation uniforms could be swift. When one nurse revoked the permit of a midwife at a conference for the renewal of permits, the nurse reported that it "was so upsetting to the midwife that long wailing sobs penetrated the air. The sympathy of the other 75 midwives brought on more sobbing—needless to say I wondered just what I'd do to restore order and continue with the meeting."[40]

Midwives also had their permits temporarily revoked if they tested positive for syphilis. Nurses kept watch over midwives' health, fearing that they would spread diseases to birthing women and infants. The nurse required the midwife to have a Wassermann test for syphilis, and vaccine against typhoid fever and smallpox.[41] Nurses administered Wassermann tests before they renewed permits each year, and nurses forbade midwives who had syphilis from performing any deliveries. If the midwife tested positive for syphilis, she had to undergo treatment and a doctor had to indicate when it was safe for her to perform deliveries again. In 1928, Nurse McDaniel reported that "the one who had a positive Wassermann is taking treatment regularly and we hope we can give her a permit before long. She asks about her permit each time she comes in."[42]

In extreme cases, health departments called on police power to force compliance with the rules. In 1931 Nurse Josie Strum of Clarke County chose to handle one midwife with extraordinary measures as a warning to all midwives. Strum indicated in her report: "Another midwife was discovered practicing midwifery without a permit, warnings did not seem to do any good so we had her arrested. She was convicted and fined. Now she is very anxious for a permit as well as several others in that same neighborhood."[43] In later years the state even used its regulatory power to punish midwives who engaged in civil rights activity. A former midwife living in Greenville in the 1960s claimed she lost her permit because she "demonstrated and sat in down at Jackson."[44]

The Midwife as Public Health Worker

Ironically, Mississippi's regulation of midwives, which limited the health services that midwives were permitted to provide, led to the creation of additional public health workers for the state. Gradually, health department officials, especially public health nurses, realized that midwives were assets in black community health work. In the early 1930s, Mississippi's executive officer of the board of health indicated that supervision, which was "primarily designed to render least harmful to the public health the services of these midwives, has converted them into important allies in the cause of human well-being."[45]

Midwives seized on the resources provided by public health nurses. They became an important conduit for health education in their childbirth work and elsewhere. They provided health instruction to adults and children through the churches and schools. The activities of midwife Mollie Gilmore of Vicksburg during 1936 and 1937 illustrate the range of midwives' health work. Gilmore accompanied the public health nurse in her home visits to mothers, and she encouraged people to go to a local church for typhoid shots. "By my influence," the midwife reported, "Dr. Smith was able to protect 80 people from typhoid fever." She gave health lectures at church and "prayed to the congregation after service." In the fall of 1936, she "talked to 100 different people on prenatal care, and health and care of the baby." She observed, "During that time I referred 5 expectant mothers to doctor." In addition, she assisted a doctor with the home deliveries of four white women, and she worked on the annual May Day child health program.[46]

Midwives provided communities with information about proper home birthing environments through model delivery room demonstrations. Beginning in the early 1930s, the board of health required that twice a year midwives set up a model room in their homes and invite their clients and other people in the community to visit. The purpose was to force the midwife to demonstrate to the public the correct birthing room, and to educate future mothers and community members about modern childbirth requirements. The delivery room was supposed to be a neatly organized, clean bedroom with newspapers spread on the floor, a paper pad placed on the bed with a drip sheet leading into a bucket, and adequate lighting and heating.[47]

These demonstrations were a clever way to ensure that midwives were familiar with state regulations, and they also provided publicity to white and black people about the state health board's work with midwives. Plantation owners, insurance agents, doctors, teachers, students, mothers, and tenant farmers all attended the delivery room demonstrations. A sizable number of midwives complied with the demonstration requirement. For example, in 1934 over 1,300 midwives sent in reports of their model delivery rooms.[48]

Midwives performed important public health work when they encouraged women to receive prenatal and postnatal care, often bringing them to the health department or mothers' clinics themselves. Retired county health officer Dr. W. E. Riecken, Jr., stated that midwives often accompanied their clients to the county health department for checkups and "frequently assisted in the exam room."[49] Midwives also aided the work of nurses by notifying them when a woman had a baby. In 1931 nurses in Sharkey and Issaquena counties reported that they "have tried to visit more lying-in cases this month but it is hard to know when they are confined. Quite a number of midwives report their cases to us right after delivery and in that way we have come in contact with more mothers during the lying-in period."[50] Midwives saw themselves as important liaisons between black communities and white health professionals. In one case in Mississippi, a midwife made requests of the local public health nurse to tend to a sick woman. In 1939 midwife Estelle W. Christian notified Nurse Viola M. Jones that a woman had come to see her at the house where she had just delivered a baby. The middle-aged woman had sores on her arms, legs, and buttocks. The midwife explained to the woman that she could not visit with the new mother or baby because she might infect them. Then the woman told the midwife that the family across the road from her had the same symptoms. The midwife wrote the nurse:

> Now could you go out there at once to see about this. I made a lecture on the 4th Sunday in August at a church at Willows, Miss. to the people about their health. . . . I advised them if they had any sores or the least suspicion they were infected with that dreaded disease syphilis to please tell some one before it is too late. So she says she heard me talk that day and when she heard I was in the neighborhood she came to tell me about it. So I advised her to stay at home until I talked with you. So if you could come out here one day I could go to their homes with you.[51]

Midwives advocated for increased care from doctors and nurses for poor women.

Midwives assisted with venereal disease control work by encouraging pregnant women and other people in the community to have their blood tested. Venereal diseases, particularly syphilis, were a major public health concern throughout the period from 1920 to 1950. Midwives proved to be quite effective in reaching people. For example, in 1944 several nurses wondered why attendance at a venereal disease clinic was suddenly increasing until they discovered that "a leader of a midwife club who had received literature on syphilis had made talks at churches, schools and in the homes. This midwife was instrumental in sending in several young girls under sixteen years of age who had infectious syphilis."[52]

As a community leader, midwife endorsement of public health projects contributed to community cooperation. Midwives assisted health department efforts to protect African-Americans against typhoid fever and diphtheria. They promoted this preventive work at their midwife club meetings, churches, and schools.[53] In 1931 Nurse Ethel B. Marsh of Adams County mentioned that her county sponsored an antidiphtheria campaign among black infants and preschool children. She explained that "the midwives in the various sections of the county are assisting by informing parents of the various stations and dates on which toxin-antitoxin will be given."[54] Elsewhere in the state, Nurse Nell E. Austin of Forrest County indicated that

> the midwives are very helpful in getting the colored people immunized against typhoid fever. At the last midwives meeting they were asked to round up all the children in their neighborhoods and bring them to the health department and have them inoculated against typhoid fever. One midwife was in the office the very next morning with fifty-five children.[55]

Parents knew and trusted their local midwives and so more readily permitted their children to participate in health programs that midwives endorsed.

Midwives not only assisted with official health department programs; they also successfully organized their own. They ran May Day programs on child health and participated in the annual Negro Health Week programs.[56] In 1935 a midwife in Smith County reported that at their May Day program "a talk was given about the care of the teeth. A few weeks later the peddler who sells extracts, spices, and tooth paste asked the leader of the midwife club what in the world had caused so many of the people in the community to buy tooth paste."[57]

Midwives were extremely proud of their health care contributions and saw themselves as part of a great health crusade. A Simpson County midwife wrote to one nurse: "yes the sisters is praying the time to hasten so they can meet you again for further instruction. They think it so grand that old as they are they can do this great work to help foster in this great battle field of deficiency."[58] One midwife even contacted the board of health, asking for official public recognition of the work performed by midwives. She pointed out that there was a Thanksgiving Day, Christmas Day, Mother's Day, and Father's Day. She said, "It look to me we could have a Midwife Day—i ben on this job sense September 1900 an my work been close to a 1,000, an i am workin in my 81 year."[59]

The Decline of Midwives

Even though individual nurses commented in their reports on the valuable public health work performed by lay midwives, the official policy of the board of health remained to ultimately eliminate the midwives. In 1948 Nurse Supervisor Lucy E. Massey instituted a retirement program, first suggested to her by county nurses, in an effort to accelerate the elimination of midwives.[60] The plan strongly encouraged the retirement of older midwives by informing them and their families that they were too old to renew their permits, and then honoring the women with ceremonies, complete with badges stating "Retired Midwife." According to the new policy, "The midwife must promise not to practice and must hand in her permit when she receives the badge."[61] From 1948 on, not only was there a policy of retiring midwives, but all new midwives had to get a physician to testify that there was a need for their services in their community before they could receive a permit.

The retirement ceremonies probably never fooled the midwives forced out of practice, but they did provide an opportunity for the nurses and people in the community to honor the women. The public health nurse usually held the event at a local church where the midwife "would sit queen for the day."[62] Sometimes people would drop money in her lap, especially women the midwife had attended. In November 1948, midwives Mollie Merrill and Josephine Franklin were honored in a retirement ceremony at St. John Methodist Church in Forrest County. According to a newspaper report of the event, "the aged pair, clad in white uniforms and caps, and clutching small American flags, sat solemnly in pink and white decorated chairs of honor, placed near the altar." The white county nurse and the black midwife club leader each offered speeches of praise for the women. Those attending sang hymns as the members of the local midwife club led a procession, "robed in white uniforms and caps, and also carrying tiny American flags." Midwives sang, read scripture, offered up prayers, and presented gifts to the retiring midwives.[63]

The number of Mississippi midwives registered with the state began to decline in the post–World War II era, in part because of state policy, but also because of other factors such as urban migration, which resulted in fewer black midwives living on the surrounding plantations. Instead of thousands of registered midwives, by 1966 only 600 midwives had permits in the state, although they still delivered 10,000 to 12,000 babies that year. By 1975 there were only 220 registered midwives who delivered about 1,000 babies. In 1982 the state had a mere 13 registered lay midwives, by which point the state no longer issued permits or held training sessions.[64]

Conclusion

Black midwives have played an important but overlooked historical role as public health workers for rural African-Americans, performing unpaid public health work for the state. In Mississippi, the community work of black midwives was vital to the success of state health programs because of their respected position and close relationship with community members. State regulation created an opportunity for midwives, long concerned with the health of their communities, to assist with state public health work. Because regulation put midwives into constant contact with public health nurses, midwives became vital assistants to nurses in implementing state health policy. From 1920 to 1950, midwives actually broadened their responsibilities for community health care, despite state regulation that set limitations on the activities of midwives. Indeed, the success of health reform in Mississippi depended on the work of women at the bottom of the medical hierarchy—black lay midwives.

Susan L. Smith, PhD
Assistant Professor of History and Women's Studies
Department of History
University of Alberta
2-28 Henry Marshall Tory Building
Edmonton, AB T6G 2H4
Canada
Phone: (403) 492-2238 (Office)
Fax: (403) 492-9125

Acknowledgments

The author would like to thank the anonymous reviewers and the following people for their support and their comments on earlier drafts of this material: Andrea Friedman, Maureen Galitski, Linda Gordon, Judith Walzer Leavitt, Gerda Lerner, Donald Macnab, Leslie Reagan, Leslie Schwalm, Mariamne Whatley, and Nancy Worcester. Special thanks to Anne Lipscomb at the Mississippi Department of Archives and History in Jackson and to Edna Roberts, retired public health nurse and former state supervisor of nursing for the Mississippi Department of Health.

This research was funded by the Woodrow Wilson National Fellowship Foundation Rural Policy Fellowship and the Women's Studies Research Grant, with additional financial assistance from the University of Wisconsin–Madison in the form of a KNAPP Women's History Fellowship Grant, the Graduate School Domestic Travel Fellowship, and the Maurice L. Richardson Fellowship from the History of Medicine Department at the University of Wisconsin Medical School.

Notes

1. This article is based on material from my dissertation, "'Sick and Tired of Being Sick and Tired': Black Women and the National Negro Health Movement, 1915–1950" (PhD diss., University of Wisconsin–Madison, 1991), chapter 5. Although not directly parallel, a similar argument has been made about the important public health role prostitutes could play in the current AIDS epidemic. Gloria Lockett, "Black Prostitutes and AIDS," in *The Black Women's Health Book: Speaking For Ourselves,* ed. Evelyn C. White (Seattle, Wash.: The Seal Press, 1990), 189–92.

2. For an excellent historiographical essay on midwives, see Judith Barrett Litoff, "Midwives and History," in *Women, Health, and Medicine in America,* ed. Rima D. Apple (New York: Garland Publishing, 1990), 443–58. On black midwives, see Molly C. Dougherty, "Southern Midwifery and Organized Health Care: Systems in Conflict," *Medical Anthropology: Cross Cultural Studies in Health and Illness* 6 (Spring 1982): 113–26; Sharon A. Robinson, "A Historical Development of Midwifery in the Black Community: 1600–1940," *Journal of Nurse-Midwifery* 29 (July/August 1984): 247–50; Linda Janet Holmes, "African American Midwives in the South," in *The American Way of Birth,* ed. Pamela S. Eakins (Philadelphia, Pa.: Temple University Press, 1986), 273–91; and Debra Anne Susie, *In the Way of Our Grandmothers: A Cultural View of Twentieth-Century Midwifery in Florida* (Athens: University of Georgia Press, 1988).

3. One must be careful not to overdraw the respect that the board of health in general, and nurses in particular, held for midwives. For example, the nursing division of the health board had a habit of collecting lists of examples of midwife illiteracy drawn from midwife club reports. Typewritten sheet of quotes, no date, box 27, Record Group 51, Mississippi Department of Health, Mississippi State Department of Archives and History (hereafter cited as MSDAH), Jackson.

4. Molly Ladd-Taylor, "Women's Health and Public Policy," in *Women, Health, and Medicine in America,* ed. Rima D. Apple (New York: Garland Publishing, 1990), 398. On the relationship between professionals and clients, see Linda Gordon, *Heroes of Their Own Lives: The Politics and History of Family Violence* (New York: Viking, 1988), especially introduction.

5. The major works on the history of lay midwifery include Frances K. Kobrin, "The American Midwife Controversy: A Crisis of Professionalization," in *Women and Health in America,* ed. Judith Walzer Leavitt (Madison: University of Wisconsin Press, 1984), 318–26; Jane B. Donegan, *Women and Men Midwives: Medicine, Morality and Misogyny in Early America* (Westport, Conn.: Greenwood Press, 1978); and Judith Barrett Litoff, *American Midwives, 1860 to the Present* (Westport, Conn.: Greenwood Press, 1978). See also Charlotte G. Borst, "Catching Babies: The Change from Midwife to Physician-Attended Childbirth in Wisconsin, 1870–1930" (PhD diss., University of Wisconsin–Madison, 1989).

6. "Percentage of births attended by physicians and midwives and others, in certain states, as reported by State Bureaus of Child Hygiene for 1925," Central File, 1925–1928, box 274, Record Group 102, U.S. Children's Bureau, National Archives (hereafter cited as NA); and Elizabeth C. Tandy, "The Health Situation of Negro

Mothers and Babies in the United States," Children's Bureau, March 1941, box 27, RG 51, MSDAH. Although my focus is on black midwives in the Southeast, specifically in Mississippi, midwives in the Southwest faced similar historical patterns.

7. See chart on white and black births in Mississippi, box 27, RG 51, MSDAH; and "The Relation of the Midwife to the State Board of Health," Mississippi State Board of Health, 1 January 1944, box 57, RG 51, MSDAH. For one midwife's accounting, see "History of Della Falkner: Mid-Wife and Register of Her Patients," published in Holly Springs, 26 February 1937, and newsclipping, "State Midwife Tells All In Booklet," 15 December 1937, box 27, RG 51, MSDAH. In the ten years from 1926 to 1936, she delivered 120 black babies and thirteen white. See also Litoff, *American Midwives,* 27; Judy Barrett Litoff, *The American Midwife Debate: A Sourcebook on Its Modern Origins* (New York: Greenwood Press, 1986), 4; and Tandy, "The Health Situation of Negro Mothers and Babies in the United States."

8. "The Relation of the Midwife to the State Board of Health," Mississippi State Board of Health, 1 January 1935, box 2, RG 51, MSDAH; Dougherty, 116–17; and Holmes, "African American Midwives in the South," 278–82. Oral interviews and autobiographical accounts of midwives illustrate these points. See Onnie Lee Logan as told to Katherine Clark, *Motherwit: An Alabama Midwife's Story* (New York: E. P. Dutton, 1989); Susie, chapter 1; and Linda Janet Holmes, "Thank You Jesus to Myself: The Life of a Traditional Black Midwife," in *The Black Women's Health Book: Speaking for Ourselves,* ed. Evelyn C. White (Seattle, Wash.: The Seal Press, 1990), 98–106. I also learned much about black midwives from Edna Roberts, a retired white public health nurse and former state supervisor of nursing in Mississippi. Edna Roberts, interview by author, tape recording, Mississippi, 17 September 1989.

9. Logan, 52; Litoff, *American Midwives,* 28; Litoff, *The American Midwife Debate,* 4; "Report on the Midwife Survey in Texas," Bureau of Child Hygiene, Texas State Board of Health, 1924, Central File, 1925–1928, box 275, RG 102, NA, and reprinted in *The American Midwife Debate,* 67–81.

10. Thordis Simonsen, ed., *You May Plow Here: The Narrative of Sara Brooks* (New York: Touchstone Books, 1986), 172.

11. Jack Bleich, "Midwife's Delivery 82 Years Ago Began Tradition for Bessie Sutton," *Jackson Clarion Ledger,* 17 September 1978, and "Grannies: The roots of midwifery," *Jackson Clarion Ledger,* 31 January 1982, both in folder-midwives, Subject File, MSDAH; and Emily Herring Wilson, *Hope and Dignity: Older Black Women of the South* (Philadelphia, Pa.: Temple University Press, 1983), 43; Holmes, "African American Midwives in the South," 280–81; and Logan, 103–4.

12. Dr. Felix J. Underwood, director of the Bureau of Child Welfare of the Mississippi State Board of Health, to Jesse O. Thomas, 3 May 1921, General Office File, box A6, Records of the National Urban League Southern Regional Division, Library of Congress.

13. Laurie Jean Reid, "The Plan of the Mississippi State Board of Health for the Supervision of Midwives," 1921 speech, box 354, RG 51, MSDAH. See also Grace L. Meigs, *Maternal Mortality from All Conditions Connected with Childbirth in the United States and Certain Other Countries,* U.S. Department of Labor, Children's Bureau Publication, No. 19 (Washington, D.C.: Government Printing Of-

fice, 1917), reprinted in Litoff, *The American Midwife Debate,* 50–66; and Litoff, *American Midwives,* 50–51, and 55.

14. Financial support came from the Sheppard–Towner Maternity and Infancy Protection Act of 1921, which provided states with federal funding for maternal and child health programs. States applied for matching grants to the U.S. Children's Bureau, which administered the act. On Mississippi, see Grace Abbott, Children's Bureau, to Governor Lee M. Russell, 12 December 1921, 1921–1924, Central File, box 249, RG 102, NA; and "Plan for the Division of Maternity and Infant Hygiene For 1922," Correspondence and Reports, 1917–1954, box 17, RG 102, NA. See also Molly Ladd-Taylor, *Raising A Baby the Government Way* (New Brunswick, N.J.: Rutgers University Press, 1986), 5–29.

15. Litoff, *The American Midwife Debate,* 5.

16. Lois Trabert, Bureau of Child Hygiene of Mississippi State Board of Health, to Dr. Anna E. Rude, Children's Bureau, 2 April 1923, Central File, 1921–1924, box 248, RG 102, NA.

17. Mary D. Osborne, "Public Health Nursing," 17 September 1938, box 317, RG 51, MSDAH.

18. Litoff, *American Midwives,* 80; and Litoff, *The American Midwife Debate.*

19. Mississippi State Board of Health, "Plan for the Division of Maternity and Infant Hygiene For 1922," 1917–1954, Correspondence and Reports, 1917–1954, box 17, RG 102, NA; Mississippi State Board of Health, "Study of Midwife Activities in Mississippi, July 1, 1921–June 30, 1929," 30 June 1929, box 36; Mississippi State Board of Health, "The Relation of the Midwife to the State Board of Health," 1 July 1937, box 356; and Mississippi State Board of Health, "The Relation of the Midwife to the State Board of Health," 1 January 1944, box 57, all in RG 51, MSDAH. See also Neil R. McMillen, *Dark Journey: Black Mississippians in the Age of Jim Crow* (Urbana: University of Illinois Press, 1989), 169.

20. Proceedings of the Negro Health Week Planning Meeting, Tuskegee, 20 January 1927, box 18, Thomas Monroe Campbell Papers, Tuskegee University. See also H. G. Perry, State Registrar of Vital Statistics, Alabama State Board of Health, to Jesse O. Thomas, 25 April 1921; and State Epidemiologist of North Carolina Board of Health to National Urban League, 12 May 1921, both letters in General Office File, box A6, National Urban League Southern Regional Division; Wilson, 39; Susie, 35; and Edward H. Beardsley, *A History of Neglect: Health Care for Blacks and Mill Workers in the Twentieth-Century South* (Knoxville: University of Tennessee Press, 1987), 39.

21. These figures should be taken merely as rough estimates. Roberts, interview by author; Dr. Felix J. Underwood, "Midwife Activities in Mississippi," [1932?], box 354; Mississippi State Board of Health, "The Relation of the Midwife to the State Board of Health," 1 July 1937, box 356; and infant and maternal mortality rates drawn from the U.S. Bureau of the Census, reported in "The Relation of the Midwife to the State Board of Health," by the Mississippi State Board of Health, 27 April 1938, box 36; U.S. Bureau of the Census, reported in "The Relation of the Midwife to the State Board of Health," by the Mississippi State Board of Health, 1 January 1944, box 57, all in RG 51, MSDAH.

22. The first midwife manual in Mississippi was published in 1922. Lois Tra-

bert, Narrative Report of Work with Midwives, June 1921 to June 1922, Central File, 1921–1924, box 248, RG 102, NA; Mississippi State Board of Health, *Manual for Midwives,* see 1928, 1939, and 1952 in box 354, and Mississippi State Board of Health, "Midwife Supervision," [1938?], box 354, all in RG 51, MSDAH. Most southern states published midwife manuals, including Georgia in 1922 and Florida beginning in 1923. See *Lessons for Midwives,* Georgia State Board of Health, Child Hygiene Publication No. 17, Prenatal Series No. 3 [1922], reprinted in Litoff, *The American Midwife Debate,* 200–207; and Susie, 241, endnote 24.

23. Dr. Felix J. Underwood, "The Development of Midwifery in Mississippi," read before the Southern Medical Association, 1925, box 36, RG 51, MSDAH; and Photo entitled "A group of midwives in Madison County before any instructions," no date, box 27, RG 51, MSDAH.

24. Quoted in Holmes, "African American Midwives in the South," 287. On midwives and birthing positions, see Laurie Jean Reid, "The Plan of the Mississippi State Board of Health for the Supervision of Midwives," 1921, box 354, RG 51, MSDAH; Litoff, *The American Midwife Debate,* 4; and Holmes, "African American Midwives in the South," 286. See also Dougherty, 117.

25. Dr. W. E. Riecken, Jr., 17 July 1990, written responses to questions posed by author. See also George Stoney, "All My Babies: Research," in *Film: Book 1,* ed. by Robert Hughes (New York: Grove Press Inc., 1959), 79–96, especially 83.

26. Nurse Elsie Davis, Holly Springs, in "Nurses Narrative Report, Mississippi State Board of Health, Bureau of Child Hygiene, Division of Public Health Nursing, July 1931," box 36, RG 51, MSDAH.

27. Nurses Abbie G. Hall and Caroline Bourg, Sharkey and Issaquena Counties, "Nurses Narrative Report, Mississippi State Board of Health, Bureau of Child Hygiene, Division of Public Health Nursing, July 1931," box 36, RG 51, MSDAH.

28. Otha Bell Jones in Itta Bena to board of health, 13 April 1938, box 27, RG 51, MSDAH. It was not unusual for midwives to keep excellent records of the births they delivered. Della Falkner kept a list of the name of every birth she attended for ten years from 1926 to 1936. "History of Della Falkner: Mid-Wife and Register of Her Patients." See also Wilson, 39.

29. Logan, 90.

30. Rosie Bell Rollins of West Point to Lucy E. Massey, 13 November 1948, box 36, RG 51, MSDAH.

31. Silver nitrate was first used for newborn's eyes in the 1870s. Susie, 4. See also Roberts, interview by author; Litoff, *American Midwives,* 101; and Litoff, *The American Midwife Debate,* 10. On midwife club reports from 1930s and 1940s, see Melissa Ann Mobley and J. E. Lucas of Carlisle Midwife Club to board of health, [1941?], midwife report for Claiborne County, 9 August 1941, and Irene B. Brisco and Louise Ceal, Humphreys County midwife club report, 5 September 1942, all in box 27; and photos of Coahoma County midwife meeting, 3 May 1951, box 21, RG 51, MSDAH. See also Mary D. Osborne to Felix J. Underwood, Narrative and Statistical Report May 1924 of the Mississippi Bureau of Child Welfare and Public Health Nursing, Central File, 1921–1924, box 249, RG 102, NA. For a discussion of midwife meetings in Florida see Susie, 46.

32. Violor Dorsy and Earline Morris of Hub to board of health, box 36;

photos of Holmes County midwife meeting, October 1938; and photos of Forrest County midwife meeting, no date, in box 27, RG 51, MSDAH. See also Dougherty, 116.

33. Lyrics to "Midwife Song: Protect the Mother and Baby" and "Song of the Midwives" sung to tune of "As We Go Marching On," box 27; and Robert Loftus, "Stork Loses Two Long-Time Forrest County Helpers," *Hattiesburg American,* 29 November 1948, box 36, RG 51, MSDAH.

34. John Lomax built a collection of black folk song recordings at the Library of Congress. *The Mississippi Doctor* 14 (June–May 1936–1937), and "Song's Recorder Here: Midwife Song Taken," newsclipping, 9 March 1937, box 36, RG 51, MSDAH. See also Dr. James Ferguson, who described a visit to a midwife meeting in October 1948 at which a phonographic recording of the entire meeting was made. James H. Ferguson, "Mississippi Midwives," *Journal of the History of Medicine* 5 (Winter 1950): 90–95, box 36, RG 51, MSDAH.

35. Nurse Agnes B. Belser and Nurse Inez Driskell, in Report from Mary D. Osborne to Dr. Felix J. Underwood, Dr. Anna E. Rude, and Dr. W. S. Leathers, September 1923, Central File, 1921–1924, box 248; and excerpts from nurses in "Narrative and Statistical Report, June 1926," Correspondence and Reports, 1917–1924, box 17, RG 102, NA.

36. Nurse Louise James, in Mississippi State Board of Health, Nursing Narrative and Statistical Report, November 1923, Central File, 1921–1924, box 249, RG 102, NA.

37. Mississippi State Board of Health, "The Relation of the Midwife to the State Board of Health," 1 July 1937, box 356; and Mississippi State Board of Health, "The Relation of the Midwife to the State Board of Health," 1 January 1944, box 57, RG 51, MSDAH.

38. Quote from Nurse Mae Reeves, in Mary D. Osborne report to Dr. Felix J. Underwood, Dr. Anna E. Rude, and Dr. W. S. Leathers, September 1923, Central File, 1921–1924, box 248, RG 102, NA.

39. Nurse report from Washington County, in Narrative and Statistical Report of the Mississippi Bureau of Child Welfare and Public Health Nursing, from Mary D. Osborne to Felix J. Underwood, May 1924, Central File, 1921–1924, box 249, RG 102, NA.

40. Zona C. Jelks, president of the Mississippi Public Health Association, "My Twenty-Five Years in Public Health in Mississippi," talk at the annual convention, 29 November 1967, box 317, RG 51, MSDAH.

41. Mississippi State Board of Health, "Midwife Supervision," [1938?], box 36, RG 51, MSDAH. Apparently, domestic servants were also required to be tested for syphilis. See Susan Tucker, *Telling Memories Among Southern Women: Domestic Workers and Their Employers in the Segregated South* (Baton Rouge: Louisiana State University Press, 1988), 177.

42. See Mississippi State Board of Health, *Manual for Midwives,* 1939, box 354, RG 51, MSDAH; and Nurse A. E. McDaniel in Tishomingso County, Mississippi State Board of Health, Bureau of Child Hygiene and Public Health Nursing, Public Health Nurses' Narrative Reports, July 1928, State Boards of Health, box 41, RG 90, United States Public Health Service (USPHS). Also see Mississippi State Board

of Health, "Study of Midwife Activities in Mississippi, July 1, 1921–June 30, 1929," 30 June 1929, box 36; and Nurse Elois Conn of Amite County, newsclipping from *Southern Herald,* 12 November [1941?], box 27, RG 51, MSDAH.

43. Nurse Josie Strum, Clarke County, "Nurses Narrative Report, Mississippi State Board of Health, Bureau of Child Hygiene, Division of Public Health Nursing, July 1931," box 36, RG 51, MSDAH.

44. Quoted in "State Health Agency Calls Midwifery 'Dying Avocation,'" newsclipping in *Jackson Commercial Appeal,* [1966?], box 36, RG 51, MSDAH.

45. Dr. Felix J. Underwood, "Midwife Activities in Mississippi," [1932?], box 354; and Mississippi Department of Health, "Policies Regarding Midwife Supervision," 1 June 1948, box 36, RG 51, MSDAH.

46. "Report of Work of Mollie Gilmore, Midwife, For July 1936 to December 1937," box 27, RG 51, MSDAH.

47. Photo of a midwife and Mrs. Robley, possibly the nurse, showing a delivery room, no date, box 21; Photo entitled "Model Midwife Delivery Room" in Sharkey County, 1953, box 36; sketch of a model delivery room, no date, box 27; and Nurse Elois Conn, newsclipping from *Southern Herald,* all in RG 51, MSDAH.

48. Mississippi State Board of Health, "The Relation of the Midwife to the State Board of Health," 1 January 1935, box 2; newsclipping entitled "Midwives and Health Work," [1933?], box 36; and Mississippi State Board of Health, "Midwife Supervision," [1938?], box 36, all in RG 51, MSDAH. See also Roberts, interview by author.

49. Dr. W. E. Riecken, Jr., written responses to author's written questions, 17 July 1990; and Ferguson, "Mississippi Midwives," 89.

50. Nurses Abbie G. Hall and Caroline Bourg, Sharkey and Issaquena Counties, "Nurses Narrative Report, Mississippi State Board of Health, Bureau of Child Hygiene, Division of Public Health Nursing, July 1931," box 36, RG 51, MSDAH.

51. Midwife Estelle W. Christian to Nurse Viola M. Jones in Claiborne County, 5 October 1939, box 27, RG 51, MSDAH.

52. Mississippi State Board of Health, "The Relation of the Midwife to the State Board of Health," 1 January 1944, box 57, RG 51, MSDAH. See also Allan M. Brandt, *No Magic Bullet: A Social History of Venereal Disease in the United States Since 1880* (New York: Oxford University Press, 1987).

53. Letter from unknown midwife in Raleigh to board of health, no date, box 27; and Nurse Fannie Mae Howell of Holmes County, "Nurses Narrative Report, Mississippi State Board of Health, Bureau of Child Hygiene, Division of Public Health Nursing, July 1931," box 36, RG 51, MSDAH.

54. Nurse Ethel B. Marsh of Adams County, "Nurses Narrative Report, Mississippi State Board of Health, Bureau of Child Hygiene, Division of Public Health Nursing, July 1931," box 36, RG 51, MSDAH.

55. Nurse Nell E. Austin of Forrest County, "Nurses Narrative Report, Mississippi State Board of Health, Bureau of Child Hygiene, Division of Public Health Nursing, July 1931," box 36, RG 51, MSDAH.

56. Mississippi State Board of Health, "The Relation of the Midwife to the State Board of Health," 1 January 1935, box 2, RG 51, MSDAH. See also Nurse Mary L. Gregory, Narrative and Statistical Report, April 1924, Mississippi State

Board of Health, Bureau of Child Hygiene and Public Health Nursing, Central File, 1921–1924, box 249, RG 102, NA.

57. Midwife leader in Smith County, quoted in "The Relation of the Midwife to the State Board of Health," Mississippi State Board of Health, 1 January 1935, box 2, RG 51, MSDAH.

58. Midwife report from Simpson County, no date but 1930s or 1940s, box 27, RG 51, MSDAH.

59. Letter from unknown midwife to board of health, no date, box 36, RG 51, MSDAH.

60. Brooksie W. Peters for the nursing staff of the Lauderdale County Health Department to Lucy E. Massey, 14 July 1947, box 36; and Dr. Andrew Hedmeg, Jackson County Health Department, reporting on nurses' suggestions to Lucy E. Massey, 8 September 1947, box 36, RG 51, MSDAH. Florida's midwife retirement efforts also began in the 1940s. Susie, 47.

61. Mississippi State Board of Health, "Policies Regarding Midwife Supervision," 1 June 1948, box 36; and memo from Lucy E. Massey to Dr. Felix J. Underwood, 2 February 1948, and memo from Dr. Felix J. Underwood to Massey, 2 February 1948, box 36, RG 51, MSDAH.

62. Roberts, interview by author.

63. Loftus, "Stork Loses Two Long-Time Forrest County Helpers."

64. By 1951 there were only about thirty white midwives. Dr. D. Galloway and Nurse Louise Holmes, Mississippi State Board of Health, to Dr. Lucille Marsh, U.S. Children's Bureau, 3 December 1951; "State Health Agency Calls Midwifery 'Dying Avocation'"; Note to Miss Ferguson on midwife figures as of December 1975, all in box 36, RG 51, MSDAH. See also "Grannies: The roots of midwifery"; Jelks, "My Twenty-Five Years in Public Health"; and Roberts, interview by author. A similar pattern held in Florida, with only a few registered midwives by the 1980s. Susie, 55.

Midwives as Wives and Mothers: Urban Midwives in the Early Twentieth Century

LINDA V. WALSH
Education Programs Associates–San Jose State University

Midwifery has been described as an occupation, a spiritual calling, and a profession. Any description of the practice has been influenced by the scholar's beliefs about health and illness, sources of knowledge, the role of the health care provider during childbirth, and the sociocultural role of women. Few historians have used feminist methods to provide new ways of seeing, and thus interpreting, midwives' lives and practices. Not until we analyze midwifery in the context of women's life experiences will we better understand the actions and influences of midwives in the changing American health care system of the early twentieth century.

Historian Elizabeth Pleck has noted that in analyzing the behaviors of family members in the home and workplace, scholars must address the question, "How did the physical and emotional demands of work alter family life?"[1] Few unskilled occupations generate demands on family outside the actual work hours that the mother is absent from the home. Professional careers, on the other hand, often place demands of time and energy on the life of family members. In this context, midwifery fits more in the category of profession or career, rather than occupation. Indeed, the European model of care to childbearing women that evolved in the twentieth century maintained the centrality of the professional midwife in the health care delivery system. However, those shaping the American system for obstetrical care excluded midwifery as an outdated and unscientific approach to childbearing women. Until recently, there has been little investigation of the midwives' actions during this dramatic change in the care available to women during their birthing experiences.

In order to better understand midwifery practice in the first three decades of this century, this research uses the "voices" of midwives, their family members, and women who hired them to identify previously over-

Nursing History Review 2 (1994): 51–65.

looked sources. Interview data was supplemented by written public records such as birth certificate data, midwife registries, and church records. Anna Carastro, a midwife in practice in Philadelphia from 1925 to 1940, provided the central voice for this article. While she speaks as an individual, additional data support her experiences and beliefs as representative of other formally urban immigrant midwives.

Economic Status of Midwives' Families

Most previous studies of immigrant working women have analyzed the work and family experiences of women in unskilled or semiskilled employment.[2] The fact that midwifery was perceived by women and communities as professional work suggests that midwives' experiences may have been different from those of women working in factories, stores, offices, or in homes. Midwives occupied positions of social status similar to that of physicians, teachers, or other professionals within the immigrant communities. One well-known, busy Philadelphia midwife, Maria Straka, saw herself professionally "like a doctor," and perceived herself as more socially privileged than other families in the neighborhood.[3] Another midwife, Salie Mackiewicz, was "like a doctor [or] nurse."[4] Anna Carastro and Rebecca Gorodetzer, both educated in university-level midwifery programs, were respected in their communities as professional practitioners.[5]

Income is often used as an indirect indicator of professional or social status. Midwives with active practices were able to attain a comfortable income from practice earnings. When a midwife maintained an active practice among the working-class families in her community, she had the ability to generate practice revenue that usually surpassed the family incomes of her patients. As one neighborhood woman recalls, "The midwives, they always had the nicest homes and their children had the best clothes."[6]

The median working woman's income in Philadelphia in 1923 was $13–$15 per week, or about $750 annually if she was able to work steadily throughout the year.[7] Full-time work throughout the year was not the norm, however, and it was not unusual for married women workers to be laid off during slow seasons.[8] In that same year, Maria Straka attended ninety-eight births and collected $1,569 in fees. A midwife who maintained a practice that averaged eight to ten births per month generated income comparable to female clerical workers, teachers, librarians, and social workers in the mid-1920s.[9] Even when a midwife with an active practice did not have additional wage earners in the household, she was able to maintain a respectable standard of living.

When a midwife maintained a fairly small practice, she usually supplemented family income in a way that facilitated attainment of the growing middle-class standard of living. Anna Carastro averaged three to four births per month in the late 1920s and early 1930s. The $750–$1,000 per year collected in fees allowed her and her husband to buy real estate and to send their children to college; eventually, Anna was able to open a licensed day nursery.

Many midwives resided in households where there were other adult wage earners. Review of the Philadelphia City Directories for the years 1915–1936 identifies numerous workers in midwife households. No doubt, most were husbands and adult children of the midwives. Occupations noted for householders indicate that the wage earners were skilled, semiprofessional, and professional workers. This finding, when compared to the occupations listed for the fathers of babies delivered by Anna Carastro and Maria Straka, suggests that the midwife households had a stronger financial base than those households of the women hiring the midwives.

In general, when householders in midwife families were identified, they occupied positions of regular, full-time employment. This was in contrast to the fathers of the infants in the birth records of Anna Carastro and Maria Straka, who typically were day laborers. Anna Carastro recalls that her husband, Mario, an ornamental ironworker, "was never a day without work. His work was in demand."[10] Rebecca Gorodetzer's husband, Meyer, made a "good living" prior to 1932 as a violinist in an orchestra and as a music teacher. The family was financially secure enough that there was always household help until the Depression.[11]

Caroline Manning, in her study of working immigrant women in Philadelphia in the 1920s, found that working mothers continued to do most of the household work necessary to maintain the family. However, she also found that it was not unusual for husbands to contribute to the efforts of housework.[12]

Practical Support in Midwife Households

Although they tended to occupy a different socioeconomic class than the working wives in Manning's study, midwives also maintained primary responsibility for the daily needs of meal preparation and child care, with husbands participating in many chores. It was not unusual for couples in working class, immigrant, and rural families to share household work while supporting each partner's outside work.[13] The concept of "separate spheres" developed by earlier historians described the development of upper-middle-class family division of labor and responsibilities, but data from other population groups suggest that the concept was not universal.[14]

Husbands of midwives often shopped, prepared meals, and provided child care to ensure that household responsibilities were assumed when midwives were called away for a case. Many Italian husbands were known for their culinary skills, particularly in the preparation of traditional pasta and "gravy."

> [My husband taught me to cook] I didn't know how to cook. My mother did everything. . . . But he learned in the service. In fact, I never did go to the butcher to buy meat. Whatever we need, he'd buy enough that during the week I didn't need to go to the store. Except for special things sometimes. But he liked to do that. I don't think it was unusual. I don't know what other people do. My mind, I'm telling you what my husband did.[15]

Other husbands completed the preparation of meals that had been planned and initiated by their wives. Maria Straka's husband, Edward, was crippled by a stroke early in his adult life but was able to get around enough to complete meals if his wife was called away. Mrs. Straka prepared food in large quantities and stored prepared dishes that needed only to be warmed in the oven. Her daughter remembers that they always had "lots of food," and that between her father and herself, complete meals were always ready at traditional mealtimes.[16]

In addition to their contributions to household help, midwives' husbands' childcare activities were essential to the smooth functioning of the family. Obviously, for those midwives whose husbands were disabled and/or not working outside the home, the constant presence of an adult family member provided stability to the children's lives. Although Maria Straka's husband could not ambulate outside the home, he was able to move around inside enough to watch the children. The children were instructed not to go outside as long as their mother was away so that they would be strictly supervised.

Able-bodied employed husbands often shifted their working schedules to accommodate their wives' work hours. Anna Carastro recalls that if she had been called away during the night, her husband would stay home from work until she returned or until he was able to find someone else to watch the children. Occasionally, their schedules did not function as smoothly as planned, and Mrs. Carastro had to take her children with her when called to a birth.

> Sometimes if there was a case, my husband was home. Sometimes I used to take the baby with me. I remember I delivered this case. I delivered the child, and this lady was from our home town. They had a fireplace in the big room upstairs. So I took the baby with me. People understood, you know. Especially because they were Italian people and they knew of me from home. The name. I didn't have any trouble.[17]

Mario Carastro sometimes took the children to the seashore for holiday while Anna Carastro stayed home because of commitments to women in the neighborhood. "And when my husband and the children went to the seashore—to Atlantic City or Wildwood—I couldn't leave because I expected some confinements. But my husband went there with the children."[18]

Older children and other relatives often helped with childcare too. With eight surviving children, there were young children who needed care in the Gorodetzer household until the late 1920s. Older siblings frequently watched Rebecca Gorodetzer's youngsters when she was called to a birth. Occasionally, relatives in the neighborhood would watch her children for short periods of time. But Mrs. Gorodetzer also had to bring one or more of her children with her on occasion when she left the house on professional business. Millie, her youngest child, remembers being taken to Polyclinic Hospital when her mother went for bag checks and renewal of her midwifery certificate. She also recalls being taken to at least one house and being watched downstairs by householders while her mother attended a laboring woman upstairs.[19]

Almarinda Cimini's household consisted of her husband and children, as well as her husband's brother, his wife, and their children. Almarinda developed a busy midwifery practice while raising three children. Her sister-in-law provided the necessary childcare for both families and assumed many of the household responsibilities while Mrs. Cimini and the two husbands worked outside the home. In this way, the families could save money while they planned the purchase of a second home.

When married, separated, or widowed working-class or poor mothers entered the workforce, they often did so only until children could begin to supplement the family income with their own wages. Studies in the 1920s indicated that once children in poor working class families were of working age, they quit school to pursue paid work.[20] The education and work history of the children of midwife mothers, however, suggests that wages of children did not become a substitute for midwife earnings. Midwives' children stayed in school and often pursued higher education. Anna Carastro's two children both went to college.

> My husband said, "My children will never go to factory work. I am the working man. My children will go to school until they have a good education." I had education myself and so I wanted our children and my husband wanted our children to go as long as they wanted to go. Nancy went to Penn State College. She graduated in journalism. Joe went to Drexel Institute.[21]

Rebecca Gorodetzer's children all pursued careers, with four of the eight becoming musicians and the others entering the business professions. Maria Straka's children graduated from high school, and her son attended Pierce Business College. He pursued a career in accounting with an international oil company, while her daughter went into retail sales.

Adult children often provided continued support to their midwife mothers, even after they married and settled in their own households. Midwives who did not write in English usually had their husbands or children complete the birth registrations and reports of births that needed to be turned in to the Midwife Inspectors. Michelina Tiano's and Anna Dlugosz's grown sons completed all of their records. Even when the midwives were skilled in completing the records in English, the children often completed them because their mothers were busy. The Gorodetzer children often completed their mother's records in order to help her finish her work.[22]

Adult sons also drove their mothers to births at night. If the adult sons did not drive or have access to a vehicle, they walked with their mothers when the midwives were called out at night.[23] Adult children of midwives also acted as interpreters for their mothers when meetings with state and city officials were necessary.[24]

In addition to support from immediate family members, midwives received practical and emotional support from relatives and friends in the neighborhood. The support of women neighbors was especially important for immigrant women who had no close female relatives in this country. Anna Carastro points out:

> Believe it or not, I never had any relatives, any blood relatives whatsoever, that came to this country. No one. I know those that were my husband's. But on my own line, there was nobody.[25]

Mrs. Carastro's transition to American life was assisted first by her husband's brothers' families in Tampa, Florida, and then by his aunt in Philadelphia. However, her relationship with his aunt never developed into one that offered support through her years as a mother and a working wife. And, although her husband felt strongly about not becoming close to neighbors, a special family-type relationship developed between the Carastros and the Scotts next door.

> We never had a close [relationship] with the other neighbors. My husband didn't like the idea of being close with the neighbors. Stayed away from everybody. [We'd] be nice, but never get chummy with the neighbors. If you get chummy with the neighbors, trouble will come. They like to know everybody else's business. We were friendly, said "Hello" day or night—but not chummy. But next door, Mrs. Scott. She was like a mother to me. She had two children—Emma and Johnny. She had married late in life and had two children and her husband died. She remained a widow.[26]

Mrs. Scott's children frequently provided childcare for Mrs. Carastro's small children.

> I remember when Nancy was a little girl, when our children were young, Johnny and Emma, brother and sister, said, "Do you have to go out so we can take care of Nancy. Joe and Nancy?" They loved the children. They would remain in their care. It pays to have good neighbors. There are people . . . who make nice things happen. Never any trouble. They were nice neighbors. And my husband was not so keen to be goody-goody with everybody. Mrs. Scott was to us like a mother and father.[27]

Community Respect for Midwives

The respect held for midwives by the women and families in their communities further facilitated practice in the early decades of the century. Women recognized those midwives with skills necessary for managing problems during labor and those midwives who maintained sterile and aseptic techniques in caring for mothers and infants. Members of the community also were aware of midwives whose techniques were poor.

Of the 959 families cared for by Maria Straka during her years of practice, half hired her for at least two births, and ninety-seven hired her for three or more births. Eighteen of those families hired Mrs. Straka for five or more births.[28] Certainly, if women did not have faith in a midwife's knowledge and skills, they would not continue to hire her to attend births.

Anna Carastro also attended births for women who had hired her previously. Generally, the families for whom she offered care had lower parities than those cared for by Maria Straka, but her birth registrations document eight families who hired her for three of more births.[29]

Addresses of families hiring both Anna Carastro and Maria Straka document that popular midwives often attended most births on neighborhood blocks. Within one small four-block area in the Gray's Ferry area, Maria Straka attended 172 births between 1919 and 1933. This was during the time that two other midwives—Maggie Scarcutty and Eva Grzybowska—lived on those blocks. Mrs. Grzybowska, a Polish midwife who advertised in the City Directory in 1910, was licensed by the state in 1914 and registered with the Philadelphia Health Department in 1930. Mrs. Scarcutty may have begun practice as Mrs. Straka's practice was declining, since she was licensed and registered in January 1931.[30]

The financial support of both Maria Straka's and Anna Carastro's practices indicates that their services were respected by their clients as professional services worthy of payment, even when the client was experiencing financial burdens. Maria Straka's financial records from 1923 to 1927 document that many families paid in installments—often in increments of $2.00 per week. The total amount in fees collected through those years indicates that families paid their bills in full, accepting their obligation to Mrs. Straka.[31] Additionally, many families continued to repay Straka for her services with gifts of fruits and vegetables, meats and poultry, wines, and money.

Midwives often received gifts from family members during religious celebrations following the births. Polish and Hungarian families supported the custom of the midwife preparing the infant for baptism or berith. During the bathing of the infant, the midwife was allowed to keep the gold pieces that relatives and friends threw into the bath water.[32]

Anna Carastro's patients usually paid for her services, although not always in cash. She recalls:

> Some people, I knew who could afford and who could not. Those who couldn't afford, what could we do? But then during August time they bring the grace of God to your house—fruits and everything that the soil produces. . . . They were honest people. They pay what they could.[33]

During the Depression, she found that people could not pay her.

> Some people did not pay. They did not have money. They were starving. [During the Depression] the midwifery—there was nothing to do. The people had no money to call the midwife.[34]

Mrs. Carastro's perception of why women who had previously hired midwives gradually moved to going to the hospital for births provides further support of the pride those women felt in hiring a midwife. The immigrant women (primarily Italian) for whom she provided care did not believe in going to doctors for their care. "They didn't go to doctors at the time. They didn't call the doctors. If I need the doctor [because of a problem with the pregnancy or labor] then I said, 'Get the doctor.' "[35] Her explanation of why women who preferred midwives to doctors reversed their position reflects her observation of the economic effect on choices made for health care. "They didn't go to the *doctor* at the time. They went to the *hospital*—for nothing! They went to hospital, and they paid nothing. Or a few dollars."[36] Other neighborhood residents and institutional reports also suggest that it was the Depression that forced women who believed in midwifery care into the hospitals. When they couldn't afford the twenty to twenty-five dollars charged by the midwife, women would attend the hospital dispensaries, where they paid only twenty-five cents per visit. They could then enter the hospital when they were in labor and pay nothing for their care if they were truly destitute.[37]

Midwives also were respected as community members who contributed to assorted community organizations and causes. Rebecca Gorodetzer was active in a variety of charitable causes. She was instrumental in coordinating efforts to care for the terminally ill during the flu epidemic of 1918 when there was no room in area hospitals for admissions. She worked closely with the staff in her children's schools and would often bring knishes or strudel to the teachers and principals. Her baking skills were renowned throughout South Philadelphia, as were her nursing and midwifery skills.

The Catholic midwives were active members of their parishes and seemed to be recognized as important members of the church community. The Diamond Jubilee Parish Souvenir Book of St. Ladislaus Church notes:

> Perhaps the best known ladies in the early period of the parish were the Polish mid-wives of Nicetown. They were Mrs. Veronika Szablewska of Rowan Street, Mrs. Anna Dlugosz of Hunting Park Avenue, and Mrs. Kazmierska of Juniata Street. They assisted at a large majority of about 5,000 births that were registered at our rectory to 1942, when the last of these mid-wives stopped her practice. Mrs. Szablewska's records show that she alone accounted for about 1,200 births up to 1930, when she retired. Mrs. Anna Dlugosz participated in even more births.[38]

In many ways, the midwife served similar functions to the parish priest. She was involved with family members through birth and death. When infants were stillborn or in danger of dying in the immediate neonatal period, she baptized them to save their souls. To a certain extent, she even heard confessions regarding issues surrounding a woman's sexuality. Midwives were given the religious and civil authority to determine paternity, and in that role, had to be highly trusted members of the community. Occasionally, the question of paternity would be investigated by the civil courts, and it appears that midwives would answer inquiries truthfully but in a way that was also protective of the women for whom they cared.

> I had a case once that went to court and I had to testify in court. I can tell you because you don't know the person and you don't know where I come from. Two ladies came to call me—was winter time. And they told me that so-and-so was in labor. So I went. She was big, sitting, but she didn't have a contraction. Well, I was supposed to go visit two patients, so I said, "I'll come back if you have contractions." She said, "Please don't leave me alone." All they knew, not to make a long story, was that the husband was in service. Therefore the pregnancy was not her husband's. She didn't want people to know. She, I presume, wanted to have some confidence with me, but there was those people. So I then understood. I said, "Look, I'm coming back. I have another

one that is giving birth." That was not the truth. That was a lie. That was to get out so that the ladies would leave. Anyhow, she gave birth when I came back and the two neighbors were there. They knew her husband was in service and she gave birth. And I didn't know all this [at the time]. Somebody must have called—I don't know. But he came a day later. He came to my house. I said, "What can I tell you? I don't know anything about [the father of the baby]." . . . When I was called to testify in court, what did I have to testify? I said, "I was called. She said she was pregnant. It was not time. I went home. Was called again. I delivered the child. I don't know any secrets."[39]

Conclusion

The demands on the midwife's time, as well as the professional energy and attention she retained when at home, certainly intruded on family members' lives. When Anna Dlugosz moved in with the laboring woman's family to provide consistent care throughout the immediate postpartum period, other family members had to absorb those responsibilities that she ordinarily assumed. When Maria Straka went from one birth to another, in addition to completing her postpartum rounds, and was away from the home for more than twenty-four hours at a time, her husband and children had to adjust their usual routines to continue the daily household rituals. And, when Anna Carastro returned home after finding a woman in the very early stage of labor, she deferred any planning for family activities, knowing she would be called out again as soon as the woman's labor progressed to a more active phase.

Because of the irregular and unpredictable hours encountered in midwifery practice, householders needed to go beyond the expected chores and responsibilities shared by many families with working mothers. Unpredictability was (and continues to be) one of the most difficult factors encountered in midwifery practice. The positive effects of personal satisfaction, personal support from loved ones, and professional support from the community and colleagues in the medical field must be strong enough in a midwife's life to balance the unpredictability of her practice. For most Philadelphia midwives with successful practices that spanned the first three decades of this century, there was support sufficient to facilitate careers that continued into their older years.

Studies of working women in the early twentieth century document that on marriage, and certainly by the birth of the first child, most women left the paid workforce and committed all their time to the roles of wife and mother. Midwives, however, followed the pattern of professional women. Midwives who had successful practices or who had invested time and finances in higher education rarely left their professions altogether. Anna Carastro never considered giving up her career when she married. She was well aware of the demands of her busy practice in Sicily, yet when asked whether her husband expected her to leave her profession and remain at home with children, she was adamant. "No. I said I would never leave my profession."[40] Rebecca Gorodetzer, too, never considered leaving her profession when she married and had children. Those midwives who trained for their practices after having children also maintained their practices, even when their social and financial status changed. Michelina Tiano, Anna Nicklas Lange, and Annie Papciak Mielinichek remarried after widowhood or divorce, and stayed in practice following the subsequent marriage. Michelina Tiano chose to keep her first married name as her professional name, rather than adopt her second husband's surname.

Evidence suggests that four factors were instrumental in facilitating ongoing midwifery practice that spanned decades. Perhaps most important was the strong personal and professional support of the spouse and/or other family members. Midwives who maintained practice while married had husbands who respected their professional role enough to balance the inconveniences of work demand and unscheduled unavailability to the family. Those husbands tended to truly accept the marriage as a partnership, perhaps believing that the social position and financial remuneration rewarded the whole family, not just the individual midwife. Older and adult children and other extended family members also needed to support the midwife's efforts in order to facilitate smooth functioning of the household.

Second, any midwife with young children required reliable childcare. Whether that care was provided by the midwife's husband, older children, mother or mother-in-law, cousin, other relative, or friend, an individual who could take care of young children—often with no notice—was necessary to allow the midwife to respond to calls at all hours of the day.

A third factor that influenced the success of ongoing practice was respect among the women in the community. The midwife depended on referrals from women for whom she had provided care. Without recognition for the knowledge and skills necessary for safe practice, in addition to the strong moral values necessary for the trust inherent in the nature of the work, midwives would not be able to maintain a practice.

Finally, successful practice depended on sufficient financial remuneration to balance the demands of the position of midwife. Many women who practiced midwifery did so because their families needed the income. If the income generated by midwifery practice was not sufficient to maintain a satisfactory status of living, an assertive, intelligent woman would seek other employment. Anna Carastro, when faced with a practice that no longer was active enough to support her professionally and financially, explored further career options and opened a licensed day nursery.

Historian Alice Kessler-Harris has noted that almost all American women have been wives at some point in their lives.[41] In this respect, the midwives practicing in urban America in the early twentieth century were no different from other American women. The sociocultural roles of wife, mother, health care practitioner, and neighbor have implied work roles that have varied in demand and effort as the views of gender roles have evolved. The balancing of multiple roles was sometimes difficult, but women committed to both career and family responsibilities were able to find that balance. Anna Carastro reflects:

> If she has that ambition [to be a wife, mother, and career woman] it's not going to be hard. Anything you do with all your heart, you don't think of the hardship. You enjoy every moment. You are thirsty or going forward for what is in your own mind. No trouble. I loved the profession, but I loved children. For, what is life without children?[42]

The Philadelphia midwives represented in this sample matured in their professional roles through the maintenance of relationships that validated them as strong, intelligent, resourceful career women. Those same relationships validated the midwives' roles in the family systems of their communities. Further analysis of the life experiences of professional women will increase our understanding of the influence of family and work culture on women's experiences in the workforce.

Linda V. Walsh, CNM, PhD
Director of Clinical Education
Education Programs Associates–San Jose State University
1 West Campbell Avenue, Bldg. D
Campbell, Calif. 95008
Phone: (408) 374-3720
Fax: (408) 374-7385

Notes

1. Elizabeth H. Pleck, "Two World's in One: Work and Family," *Journal of Social History* 10 (1976–1977): 187 (hereafter cited as *JSH*).

2. For analysis of immigrant women's experiences in the United States, see Carol Groneman, "Working-Class Immigrant Women in Mid-Nineteenth Century New York: The Irish Women's Experience," *Journal of Urban History* 4 (1978): 255 (hereafter cited as *JUH*); Tamara K. Hareven, "The Laborers of Manchester, NH, 1912–1922: The Role of Family and Ethnicity in Adjustment to Industrial Life," *Labor History* 16 (1975): 249; Corinne Azen Krause, "Urbanization without Breakdown: Italian, Jewish and Slavic Immigrant Women in Pittsburgh, 1900–1945," *JUH* 4 (1978): 291; Elizabeth H. Pleck, "Two World's in One," 178; Elizabeth H. Pleck, "A Mother's Wages: Income Earning Among Married Italian and Black Women, 1896–1911," in *The American Family in Social-Historical Perspective,* 2nd ed., ed. Michael Gordon (New York: St. Martin's Press, 1978); Diane C. Vecchio, "Italian Women in Industry: The Shoe Workers of Endicott, NY 1914–1935," *Journal of American Ethnic History* 8 (1989): 60; Janice Reit Webster, "Domestication and Americanization: Scandinavian Women in Seattle, 1888–1900," *JUH* 4 (1978): 275.

3. Interview with Mary Harvey, 30 January 1989.

4. Interview with Edward Wojcik, 31 October 1989.

5. Millie Imber-Rutko, personal letter; phone interview with Harry Gorodetzer, 4 October 1988; phone interview with Michael Gorodetzer, 3 November 1988; interview with Anna Carastro, 7 April 1989.

6. Interview with Frances Suder, 6 January 1989.

7. Caroline Manning, *The Immigrant Woman and Her Job,* United States Department of Labor, Women's Bureau Bulletin No. 74 (Washington, D.C.: Government Printing Office, 1930).

8. See Louise Odencrantz, *Italian Women in Industry* (New York: ARNO Press, 1977).

9. G. E. Manson, "Occupational Interests and Personality Requirements of Women in Business and the Professions," *Michigan Business Studies* III (April 1931).

10. Interview with Anna Carastro, 9 October 1989.

11. Millie Imber-Rutko, personal letter.

12. Manning, *The Immigrant Woman.*

13. For discussion of shared household responsibilities, see Pleck, "Two Worlds in One."

14. For example, see Nancy Cott, *The Bonds of Womanhood: Women's Sphere in New England, 1780–1835* (New Haven: Yale University Press, 1977).

15. Interview with Anna Carastro, 9 October 1989.

16. Interview with Mary Harvey, 29 January 1989.

17. Interview with Anna Carastro, 7 April 1989.

18. Ibid.

19. Millie Imber-Rutko, personal letter.

20. See U.S. Congress, *Report on Condition of Woman and Child Wage Earners in the United States,* Vol 2 (Washington, D.C.: Government Printing Office, 1910);

Elyce J. Rotella, *From Home to Office: U.S. Women at Work, 1870–1930* (Ann Arbor, Mich.: UMI Research Press, 1981); Gwendolyn S. Hughes, *Mothers in Industry: Wage-Earning by Mothers in Philadelphia* (New York: New Republic, Inc., 1925); Manning, *Immigrant Women.*

21. Interview with Anna Carastro, 9 October 1989.

22. Interviews with Charles Carpino, 12 October 1988; Ann Rakszawski, 21 August 1989; Elizabeth Wolf, 9 January 1989.

23. Interviews with Charles Carpino, 12 October 1988; Harry Gorodetzer, 4 October 1988.

24. Minutes, Bureau of Medical Education and Licensure, Pennsylvania State Archives, 4 February 1921.

25. Interview with Anna Carastro, 9 October 1989.

26. Ibid., 10 October 1989.

27. Ibid.

28. Maria Straka, Birth Records.

29. Anna Carastro, Birth Records.

30. Maria Straka, Birth Records; Midwife Register, Philadelphia Department of Health, Philadelphia City Archives.

31. Maria Straka, Family Papers.

32. This custom was discussed in interviews with Anna Carastro, 7 April 1989; Mary Harvey, 30 January 1989; Harry Gorodetzer, 4 October 1988; Millie Imber-Rutko, personal letter.

33. Interview with Anna Carastro, 7 April 1989.

34. Ibid.

35. Ibid., 8 April 1989.

36. Ibid.

37. The Annual Report of Pennsylvania Hospital, 1935, addresses the fact that the institution provided free care to increasing numbers of individuals during the first five years of the Depression. Also, interviews with Ella Ruggerio, 9 November 1988, and Edward Wojcik, 31 October 1989, identified the belief that women no longer were able to pay a midwife and so sought cheaper or free care through the dispensaries and lying-in wards of the city hospitals.

38. Diamond Jubilee Parish Souvenir Book, St. Ladislaus Roman Catholic Church, Philadelphia, Pa., p. 75.

39. Interview with Anna Carastro, 7 April 1989.

40. Interview with Anna Carastro, 8 October 1989.

41. Alice Kessler-Harris, *Women Have Always Worked: A Historical Overview* (Old Westbury, N.Y.: Feminist Press, 1981).

42. Interview with Anna Carastro, 8 October 1989.

Jane A. Delano: Saint or Sellout?

RUTH E. MALONE
School of Nursing
University of California, San Francisco

> History tends to make us humble. It many times shows us that the work which we think original is only a repetition of that which has been done before. It shows us how our predecessors struggled with problems almost exactly like those we meet.
>
> Goodnow (1937)[1]

Jane A. Delano was called "the Florence Nightingale of America" for her work during a yellow fever outbreak.[2] "One of the commanding figures in American nursing," she volunteered her full-time services to the American Red Cross for the last ten years of her life; she also fought successfully to increase pay and status for military nurses.[3] During the turbulent years of World War I, she was undoubtedly the most widely beloved nurse in the United States. After her death, thousands attended memorial services held in her honor throughout the country; New York's Carnegie Hall was filled to capacity for one such service.[4] Buried with full honors at Arlington National Cemetery, she was revered, decades after her death, as a martyred heroine. Yet, at the zenith of her distinguished career, she took the side of a hospital administrator-physician against the nation's most influential nursing education leaders in a bitter "feud" over the use of aides to meet a nursing shortage—and she lost.

Why would Delano, a respected graduate of Bellevue and former president of the American Nurses' Association, take a stance that put her publicly at odds with nursing leaders such as Annie Goodrich and M. Adelaide Nutting? I will argue that Delano's decision had much to do with her upbringing and personality, her early professional experiences, her leadership style, and her grasp of the particular situation. But the three primary players in this crisis in which, as one observer put it, "the nursing profession . . . stood at the crossroads," also epitomized conflicting values that continue within nursing to this day.[5] This article will examine the World

Nursing History Review 2 (1994): 67–97.

War I aide crisis that "caused a rift in the nursing group such as no other issue had ever caused. . . . [S]o strong was the impression made upon nurses that the controversy was still fresh in the memories of many when the Second World War began."[6]

World War I, according to one account, "marks the great divide of modern times. Like a vast geological fault, it transformed a whole landscape. Nothing was untouched, from politics and economics to social relations and the arts."[7] For nursing, the war provided an opportunity to prove the value of professional training and discipline; as we shall see, it also posed a threat to professional nursing's hard-one status. Jane Delano, as director of Red Cross Nursing Service, was charged with meeting the needs for additional nurses for the military and for domestic emergencies.

Although the United States did not enter the war until 1917, the Red Cross had begun sending supplies to Europe as early as 1914. Goodnow recalled that "at the beginning no one thought of more than a few months of war . . . as country after country was drawn into the conflict the work grew so stupendous that the nursing resources of the world were taxed to their utmost."[8] In this climate of urgency, the old aide question resurfaced again.

The aide question had first arisen in 1912 when a plan had been developed to create Red Cross voluntary nursing aide detachments similar to groups then active in England—a plan headed by Marion Oliver, an enthusiastic laywoman. The plan had been vigorously opposed by organized professional nurses, including Delano, who later reminded these same nurses that at the time she "felt that our nursing standards were absolutely threatened, that our Nursing Service would be of no avail with these groups of women unrelated to us, organized by physicians, taught by physicians, serving under their guidance . . . that our nursing standards might all go by the board."[9] These standards, and nursing's right to establish them for itself, had been hard-won. Isabel Hampton had observed in 1893 that "a 'trained nurse' may mean . . . anything, everything, or next to nothing," and nursing's professional leaders had fought many battles in the intervening years to establish standards for practitioners and training schools.[10] For Delano, the critical issue was one of consolidating professional nursing's position as the authority over nursing-related personnel and activities in the Red Cross. She had threatened to resign over the aide plan:

> I told the Red Cross that if this [the voluntary aide] plan were put through that I should at once sever my connection with the Red Cross; that I believed every

member of the National Committee and every member of the State and Local Committees would go out with me.[11]

Red Cross officials knew this was no idle threat; Delano had built a loyal following among nurses and was well respected as a caring and devoted administrator. While she was not a close confidante of professional nursing leaders, they had come to count on her as their representative in the Red Cross, and clinical nurses at all levels admired her. Delano's style of leadership, built on experiences as superintendent of nurses at the University of Pennsylvania Hospital and at Bellevue, was based on a kind of maternal ideal. At Bellevue, she "forbid all training school employees to speak of the students as 'the girls,' always substituting 'the nurses,'" and she had instituted social parties and had sent graduating nurses to the opera, practices that were considered shockingly liberal at a time when rigid discipline was emphasized. She took a personal interest in her students and subordinates. "You always felt that she backed you to the limit," an associate later wrote.[12] Care, in Delano's eyes, was always paramount. "If something must be left undone," Delano told her head nurses, "let the ward look a little untidy, but make the patients comfortable."[13]

Another anecdote illustrates her nurturing style of leadership. In 1900, Delano had assumed a position as superintendent of the Girl's Department of the House of Refuge on Randall's Island, New York. This grim institution cared for "wayward girls," and a biographer later reported that Delano responded forcefully to a discussion of punishment for the girls, asserting, "I don't believe in any force but a spiritual force. If I can make these girls see what my ideals are and help me willingly to get them into this place, then I will stay and try it out. But if I am expected to control them by severity and punishment, I am ready to leave."[14]

True to her word, Delano had rented rooms in New York where she held weekly meetings for small groups of girls and made supper for them, "at the same time teaching them simple housewifely ways."[15] Strongly religious, but open-minded, she believed in setting an example and expecting the best of those who worked under her, an attitude that inspired fervent devotion and intense loyalty. Red Cross officials quickly recognized the enormous rift they would create by losing her. The Oliver aide plan was dropped, and the Red Cross Nursing Service took over development of the auxiliary nursing service, in full cooperation with the National Committee on Red Cross Nursing Service, which included representatives of the national nursing organizations.

"Formidable Subjects"

Throughout 1911, Delano had collected ideas for a course that later became "Elementary Hygiene and Home Care of the Sick," which was offered to select groups of women to "prepare them to render emergency assistance in case of accident, to give more intelligent care to their own families . . . and in exceptional cases, to assist in relief work under the supervision of the Nursing Service of the American Red Cross."[16] With Isabel McIsaac she developed the instruction book for the course. The course's purpose, according to the authors, was to "furnish some light upon those formidable subjects which lie so near to the lives of housemothers, whose labors for untold ages have been obscured by the idea that little intelligence is required to keep house and care for a family."[17]

Despite the misgivings of many graduate nurses, who feared that the laywomen taking the course would then consider themselves to be nurses (a concern that Delano and McIsaac attempted to address by eliminating the word "nursing" from the title of the book), the course proved a popular one in the pro–public health climate of the time. Instructed only by carefully screened graduate nurses, who were cautioned not to permit any confession between the roles of professional and amateur nurse, the courses were received enthusiastically. In 1914, the Red Cross issued 273 certificates of completion for the course; by 1918, 27,942 certificates were issued for the year; and in 1920, 117,908 completed the course.[18] But the very success of these courses created a body of women who clamored for service in the frenzied patriotism of the war years. Delano herself had been anxious about such a prospect; she had helped persuade Clara Noyes to join her in Red Cross work in a 7 June 1916 letter, in which she suggested that "there is a distinct menace to our nursing standards in the development of this lay personnel unless it is carefully directed and supervised."[19] But Delano could hardly have foreseen the scope of the problems that lay ahead.

During the early war years, Delano and her Red Cross nursing office staff, which grew as the war needs became more pressing, had performed a masterful organizational feat: enrolling thousands of nurses through a laborious process of checking references and schools, writing to superintendents, sending nurses to various domestic emergencies, and developing the programs aimed at lay volunteers. Busy though she was, Delano made a point of trying to see off groups of nurses as they sailed for Europe, taking intense personal interest in their welfare. Dock and her colleagues detail the Christmas boxes filled with cocoa, coffee, soap, chocolate, and sweaters that

Delano put together with her own money to send to "her lambs" overseas.[20] Delano wrote to a Miss Krueger:

> I am more than grieved to hear of your illness and that of the other nurses at Gevgeli and am so worried for fear you are not able to get any kind of suitable food. Were it not for the fear that there would not be enough nurses to take care of those who are ill, I should not send other nurses into this danger.[21]

Conditions were often deplorable. An American woman who volunteered in a French army hospital wrote home: "When I tell you that I have one large needle for my whole Pavilion, and that I am obliged to give an average of fifteen injections a day with it—and as if that were not enough, the doctor frequently asks to borrow it for another hospital—you may guess how it all goes."[22]

Beginning around 1916, the Red Cross organized base hospital medical teams, some of which were dispatched to assist in European countries already involved in the war. At the request of the War Department, it was decided to organize groups of twenty-five nurses' aides to accompany each 100-nurse base hospital unit, each aide being required to complete the home care course plus one month's hospital training.[23] As the war situation intensified, and particularly after the United States entered the war, hundreds of women of various levels of training who wanted to volunteer as "nurses" swamped the Red Cross offices with their urgent requests. Historian Portia B. Kernodle quotes from a letter written by Clara Noyes to Adelaide Nutting on 8 April 1917:

> Tell Anne of Albany [Annie Goodrich] that if I were not convinced before I should be now that the most vital thing in the life of our profession is the protection of the word "nurse." Everyone seems to have gone mad. I talk until I am hoarse, dictating letters to doctors and women who want to be Red Cross nurses in a few minutes.[24]

Increasing Demands

Yet the demand for nurses was increasing apace. As graduate nurses in increasing numbers left their posts in training schools to enroll for Red Cross or military service, civil hospital authorities began to become alarmed. At this time, the nursing staff of hospitals was almost entirely composed of "pupil nurses," students in the hospital-based training programs who cared for patients under the (usually minimal) supervision of a graduate nurse.

The departure of those graduates threatened the training schools' ability to supervise the pupils so necessary to the economic and clinical functioning of the hospitals with which the schools were associated (most pupil nurses were paid a rather minimal allowance during their training).

Some administrators, such as Dr. S. S. Goldwater, administrator of New York's Mt. Sinai Hospital, seized on the situation to urge the use of aides in civilian hospitals during the crisis, an idea that clearly threatened the hard-won gains of "trained nurses."[25] Professional nursing leaders, who had struggled to convince the public of the value of nurse training, now saw before them the spectre of a return to hospitals staffed by poorly trained aides over whom professional nurses had no control. They also worried that opening paid positions to aides would decrease interest in nursing school enrollment and that aides with hospital experience would then try to pass as nurses. Since there was no national system of required registration in place, such fears were not ungrounded.

The National Committee on Red Cross Nursing Service, of which both Delano and Nutting were members, recommended in April 1917 that Red Cross aide courses be instituted to help supply base hospital units then being readied for overseas work. By late 1917, about 1,500 aides had been so trained by the Red Cross. But in June the National Emergency Committee on Nursing was formed, which later became the National Committee on Nursing of the Council of National Defense—known at the time as "Miss Nutting's committee." As Kernodle observed,

> If the main concern of the Red Cross was to enroll for military service as many as possible of the nurses already trained, the chief aim of the government committee [Miss Nutting's] was to ensure present care in civilian hospitals and a future supply of nurses both for military and civilian use. The method chosen was to expand the schools of nursing and fill them to capacity. The committee was pledged to war on short courses and to safeguarding standards of nursing and nursing education in every possible way.[26]

To that end Nutting's committee had emphasized, in a report of the 10 November 1917 meeting, that there was no need for aides. In a postscript to the minutes, the committee also deplored the "misguided" uses of aides about which they had already heard: "These young aids have been invited to assist in the operating room, have visited autopsies, and have been given responsible and unsuitable duties."[27] (There was, however, a minority view represented on Nutting's committee—that of S. S. Goldwater.)[28] Nutting's committee, the formative meeting of which Delano was unable to may have been intended to lend support to Delano's efforts to uphold nursing standards. But the proliferation of committees, many of which included the same people in various power relationships with one another, may have also contributed to the confusion regarding the aide question.

The Players in the Aide Crisis

The women who figured prominently in the aide crisis each graduated from one of what were considered the "elite" nursing schools: Jane Delano (Bellevue, 1886), Adelaide Nutting (Johns Hopkins, 1891), and Annie Goodrich (New York Hospital, 1892).[29] In addition, they all worked as superintendents of one or more of these same schools, often within a relatively short time (by today's standards) after graduating, and frequently following on one another's heels as they moved from one prestigious position to another. Annie Goodrich, for example, had followed Delano as superintendent of the training school at Bellevue; both served as president of the American Nurses' Association. Goodrich worked at Teachers College with Nutting. All three served on several committees together, and all three shared the special status reserved for a small proportion of nursing school graduates.[30] Most of this career-oriented group shared common professional values.[31] But Delano, while working closely with the other two leaders in professional nursing for many years, maintained a certain personal reservedness. As Sarah Pickett would later write in "The European War":

> She had always been a silent woman, talking little to her sister nurses regarding her hopes and plans. Among them, however, a strong fraternal spirit of inter-reliance and confidence had developed; pioneers all of them and intensely eager, they had shared their hopes and the stories of their struggles with each other, but Miss Delano had never taken them fully into her confidence. Because they did not know her well . . . they distrusted her to some extent.[32]

Annie Goodrich, who in 1917 was director of Lillian Wald's Henry Street Settlement House, a faculty member at Adelaide Nutting's Teachers College, and president of the American Nurses' Association, did not shrink from power struggles and had been drawn to nursing for reasons very different from the missionary ideals that had attracted Delano.[33] According to one biographer who knew her in later life, she was "a feminine 'Old Hickory,'" born into a wealthy family, who chose nursing after her family met with financial difficulties in 1890. She

> was quite honest with herself and admitted that she did not like nursing—far from it. She hated sickness and had a horror of death; nevertheless, since few vocational fields were open to women at that time, she decided that entering the nursing profession was the best way to solve her problem.[34]

Goodrich had wanted to go to Bellevue, but her mother discouraged this because of Bellevue's charity status, so she went instead to New York Hospital, where Lillian Wald was her student head nurse. Her organizational abilities were quickly recognized, and she advanced rapidly. But she "shrank from suffering," according to another biographer, in contrast to Delano, who seemed drawn to the downtrodden.[35] "Certainly," noted one biographer, "she [Goodrich] is not among those who definitely 'felt the call' to nursing."[36] Isabel Stewart would later describe Goodrich as "temperamental, but brilliant. She couldn't work under anyone. She had to be the top."[37] This characteristic was revealed when a curious turn of circumstances involved her deeply in the ongoing aide question and in an open battle with Delano over its resolution.

Seeds of Conflict

On 10 July 1917, according to Dock and colleagues in *History of American Red Cross Nursing,* Major Grayson Murphy, the American Red Cross representative in Europe, requested that Delano select "a trained nurse to act as head of our nursing activities in France. This woman is needed immediately." On 18 July, Delano wrote to Murphy introducing Martha Russell, and Russell sailed for France on 21 July. Meanwhile, several shifts in personnel were taking place at Red Cross National Headquarters, and Major Winford Smith was reassigned as assistant director general of Military Relief. After hours on 20 July 1917, according to Dock's account, Smith received a cable in which Dr. Alexander Lambert, liaison officer between the American Expeditionary Forces in France and the American Red Cross, specifically requested Annie Goodrich for the nursing position Delano had already assigned to Russell. Without discussing the matter with Delano, Smith sent a copy of the cable to Goodrich, who happened to be out of town. Over the next few days, during routine conferences with Delano's associate Clara Noyes, Smith learned that Russell had been sent for the position, but he failed to mention the Goodrich cable.[38]

Goodrich replied to Smith on 24 July, confirming that she had heard that Russell had assumed the position and that the matter was closed. One may surmise, however, that she may have thought that, despite the specific request for her services, Delano had selected someone else instead. This might have been the end of the matter, but things did not go well in France for Martha Russell, and at a meeting of the National Committee in October 1917, someone asked why Goodrich had not been sent instead since she had been requested. According to Dock and colleagues, "Miss Delano and Miss Noyes looked at each other in blank bewilderment" until Lillian Wald clarified the situation.[39]

It was a matter of some political embarrassment for Delano to find "that nurses outside the Red Cross organization should have known more about Red Cross administrative correspondence than did they," but in an apparent attempt to salvage the situation, Delano wrote Goodrich on 20 November and asked her if she would go to France as chief nurse for the Red Cross.[40] Several weeks later Goodrich replied with rather severe formality: "I cannot feel that I should be justified in severing lines of work, the important bearing of which on the present situation I do not believe I exaggerate, to assume for an indefinite period the work in France as you present it in your letter."[41]

Instead, Goodrich suggested, she would be willing to conduct a major survey of the nursing situation in both military and Red Cross hospitals in France, as well as in the public health arena. Since military hospitals were outside the purview of the Red Cross, Delano had no authority to engage Goodrich for such an assignment, but following yet another urgent cable from France requesting that Goodrich be sent, Delano sent to Charles E. Scott, general manager at Red Cross National Headquarters, a copy of Goodrich's letter. She added a memorandum, dated 9 January 1918:

> Some time ago I requested Miss Goodrich to accept service in France as the representative of the American Red Cross Department of Nursing. At the time she stated to me that if she were to go she would not wish to assume Miss Russell's responsibilities and should desire that either she or someone else remain in the Paris office. She expressed herself as willing to go over to make a survey of the nursing situation generally, including the military hospitals. I requested Miss Goodrich to send me a statement in regard to the matter and am sending with this her letter. I have conferred with Dr. Ward and Mr. Swan concerning the duties required of the representative of the United States in Paris, and they both agreed that supervision or inspection of the nursing service *in military hospitals* was not contemplated. . . . Under these circumstances and in view of Miss Goodrich's evident unwillingness to go to France

> for Red Cross work alone, I would suggest that a cable be sent, stating Miss Goodrich's position in the matter.[42]

Three days later, she wrote to Goodrich:

> It does not seem desirable at this time for the Red Cross to ask the Surgeon General's office to confer upon their representative in France definite authority in regard to the military hospitals.
>
> I greatly regret that you do not feel justified in going to Europe for the Red Cross alone, but the members of the commission who have recently been here assure me that the duties which they have in mind for this position do not involve any authority in connection with the military hospitals and that any attempt to secure such authority would probably not be acceptable.[43]

A week later, Dr. Lambert cabled Goodrich personally, asking again for her services and requesting a personal response. She replied that she had expressed her willingness to go under her terms, and shortly thereafter wrote to Delano again as follows:

> A message has come from the other side that seems to indicate that my services are still desired. I am loath indeed to refuse to go, but I am also firmly convinced that I can only effectively render the service they have in mind through a governmental recognition that will clearly define my position and make my opinions in matters relative to nursing authoritative. I appreciate that this is a great deal to ask, but I believe that my experience in nursing, the importance of the work I shall be asked to relinquish, and, above all, the problems I may be called upon to solve, justify this request.[44]

The Traditionalist

Delano's reluctance to push for the extension of such authority to Goodrich may have stemmed from several sources. First, though she was a strong supporter of professional standards, Delano's nursing ideals fell heavily within what Barbara Melosh, in *The Physician's Hand,* has called the "traditionalist" view.[45] This ideology, prevalent in the nineteenth century, suggested that women were naturally suited to work such as nursing by virtue of certain innately feminine characteristics, including selflessness, moral skills, and motherliness. An editorial in 1900 argued that

> the first qualification of the trained nurse should be womanliness . . . a wide and tender humanity. . . . It is a stronger emphasis on the emotional, religious,

> and humane side of her calling that the trained nurse needs today rather than a wider acquaintance with mere science.[46]

Such a view, linked to women's domestic roles within the family and group, tended to include all women, and Delano revealed these traditionalist roots at the National League for Nursing Education's Twenty-fourth Annual Convention in 1918:

> I will not take part in anything that eliminates absolutely the women of this country whose loved ones are serving in France. I believe that they have the right to share with us in the care of the men they have borne. . . . A woman came the other day, a woman past forty. Her husband had been an Army officer and he died. She had one son at the front. . . . And she talked to me and she said, "I can't take care of my own boy but is there any place I can go and do something for the boy of some other mother?" . . . We are all women. I do not think we are rich and poor, and bound and free, and all the rest of it; we are all women.[47]

Additionally, Delano could not but have been somewhat affronted by Goodrich's refusal to give her all for the cause of the Red Cross. She once confided to a friend that "the Red Cross is a religion to me"; Goodrich's demands may, therefore, have struck her as unduly self-promoting in an atmosphere in which so many sacrifices were being made by others.[48] Delano herself was a volunteer; having inherited a fortune from a wealthy benefactor who admired her self-effacing work, she declined to accept any pay for her work in the last ten years of her life.[49]

Finally, Delano was a pragmatic leader who knew how to choose her battles. Much earlier in her life, when one of her girlhood friends who had gone to nursing school wrote her to complain about the strict discipline of her training institution, Delano's answer had been plainspoken: "Take up nobody's quarrels, not even your own; stay on the fence if you die for it. After all, you are there for your training, not to run the hospital."[50] Her position at the Red Cross required her to tread a difficult and uncharted path amid the twin male-dominated hierarchies of medicine and the military; the female-dominated hierarchy of emerging professional nurses; the interests of wealthy philanthropic women, whose assistance had been invaluable to nurses in establishing professional schools and standards; the lay public; and the Red Cross itself, whose tradition carried a commitment to volunteerism. Her goal was to "stay on the fence"; she was not a revolutionary, but a reformer, and her style was to seek consensus rather than confrontation.

The Professionalists

In contrast, Goodrich clearly stands more closely aligned with the "professionalist" ideology that was gaining ground as the century turned. Susan Armeny points out that organized nurses during the early years of the twentieth century tended to align themselves with professional men rather than with women as a group.[51] Armeny contrasts the "sanitary ideal," a complex of ideas embracing organization, discipline, hierarchical relationships based on birth or training, and efficiency, with "social feminism," a traditionalist ideology of female solidarity grounded in notions of altruism, social justice, and the replication of home and family in the society as a whole. For Goodrich and other nursing "professionalists," social feminism held hidden dangers, its emphasis on domesticity and inclusiveness a direct affront to their assertions that nurses' training was important and valuable and that merely being female was not sufficient preparation for being a nurse. Professionalists were often on the defensive. Responding to a *New York Medical Journal* article that had reportedly asserted that "Nursing is an honorable, a remunerative, a noble calling, but efforts to exalt it into a profession . . . are the apotheosis of the absurd," a nurse reminded readers that

> the medical profession did not take kindly to the training of women for nurses, and it was only after hard work and the overcoming of many obstacles, after the nurse had established order and cleanliness in the hospitals and after the physicians had discovered that the percentage of deaths decreased and the percentage of recoveries increased, that they could look with favor upon her.[52]

Delano apparently made no further response to Goodrich, but Goodrich herself had perhaps decided to pursue other avenues toward her goal, for a letter from Surgeon General William C. Gorgas to the Secretary of War, dated 30 January 1918, noted that Goodrich's mentor and associate Lillian Wald had approached Gorgas with the suggestion that Goodrich be sent to Europe. Gorgas, however, felt that Goodrich might be "more valuable in this office than abroad" and suggested that she be assigned as inspector "of all hospitals to which nurses are assigned," precisely the position Goodrich desired—a position that would give her enormous influence over national nursing-policy decisions.[53]

It would appear that Nutting and Goodrich, who had been heavily involved in promoting a summer preparatory program for nurses at Vassar College and were very possibly already thinking about the prospects for an

Army School of Nursing, thus managed a kind of "end run" around the Red Cross, whose ongoing plans for the use of aides were of increasing concern to them. A telegram from Ella P. Crandall to Nutting dated 30 January confides that the Gorgas action on Goodrich was promptly approved by the Executive Committee of the General Medical Board, and on 15 February, (now) Colonel Winford Smith, who was by then in charge of the Base Hospital Division of the Surgeon General's office, wrote to advise Nutting that Goodrich's appointment as inspector of hospitals could now be made public.[54] This suggests that Nutting was involved in the behind-the-scenes maneuvering that secured such a powerful position for Goodrich.

"Aids Are Upon Us!"

On assuming her duties in Gorgas's office 18 February 1918, however, Goodrich was horrified to learn that a mere nine days previously Gorgas had notified the Red Cross to proceed with a plan to use nurses' aides as civilian employees at military hospitals, paying them thirty dollars a month plus room, board, and traveling expenses.[55] This represented a serious competitive threat to professional nurses, since pupil nurses at this time were usually paid only about ten dollars a week. She lost no time in letting Nutting know about the situation. In a handwritten letter she wrote, "The *aids* are upon us! . . . I should not have known about this had it not been for Miss Gardner. . . . I told Miss Delano that I thought this might kill the Vassar project. . . . I spent 3–5 hours with Miss Delano—I don't know how she feels this evening but I am as limp as a rag."[56]

Nutting sent both a letter and a telegram to Delano immediately, in which she emphasized, almost petulantly, that she was "very greatly disturbed over proposition to pay aids. Nurses of country will look to you to oppose it successfully. If carried out will injure work of hospitals and/or schools all over country. Incidentally we might as well advise Vassar to abandon plans for summer school."[57]

To Goodrich the next day, Nutting wrote, "we were all thoroughly depressed over the situation in Washington, and the results which we felt would certainly follow the inauguration of paid aids in the hospital service."[58] The Vassar project, to which they referred, was an ambitious attempt to stimulate interest in nursing, and it was dear to the hearts of the leaders in nursing education, who had visions of college-educated nurses.

panded three-year programs); and organizing schools for "practical training" at camp and base hospitals (threatening to legitimize health care workers who were not professional nurses). Alluding to Nutting and Goodrich, among others, he suggested that a "representative medical organization" should offer suggestions and that a committee of nurses should be appointed "who will develop it [his proposed program] rather than obstruct it."[65]

The aide conflict came to a head at the convention of the national nursing organizations in Cleveland, 7–11 May 1918. Dr. J. E. Cutler, Professor of Sociology at Western Reserve University, began the Wednesday evening meeting with a speech in which, perhaps prescient of the conflict that was to unfold, he reminded the group that

> it is difficult at a time like this to get any perspective of our tasks and responsibilities. We are overwhelmed by the multitude of adjustments that we are compelled to make all at once. . . . Our fixed habits of thinking are under attack. . . . If we are to emerge from our difficulties at the present moment, we must divest ourselves of much that has become fixed in our ways of thinking and of doing things.[66]

Cutler went on to forecast the closure of hospital schools and a four-year university program for nursing education, possibly with an option after two years of study to do private duty as a lesser-grade nurse, admitting that the idea was "only a dream."

He was followed at the podium by Adelaide Nutting, who admitted that, earlier, "probably very few of us saw clearly" what should be done, but that restricting aide courses to the Red Cross seemed preferable to a variety of short courses purporting to train aides. "I think," she emphasized optimistically, "that the nurses of this country have made a worthy record. . . . In so far as meeting the needs of the army are concerned they have been on the whole far ahead of the need."[67]

Dr. Goldwater spoke next, presenting his views on "The Nursing Crisis," which he later reprinted in the June issue of *The Modern Hospital*. Goldwater had become, over several months of intense discussions, the chief spokesman from the civil hospital community to argue for the use of aides. Civil hospital authorities were concerned about their economic future and saw volunteer, unpaid aides as a solution to their labor needs in the face of competition from paid positions in government and military service.[68] Goldwater, a physician, was an ambitious and well-connected executive who liked to take charge, and he gloried in meticulous organization.

Chairman of the Committee on Hospitals, General Medical Board, Council of National Defense, and an influential past president of the American Hospital Association, he represented interests that were many times at odds with those of professional nursing leaders.[69] In what can only be interpreted as an allusion to previous disagreements they had shared, probably as members of Nutting's committee, he began by saying, in relation to Nutting, "I am very glad that the great teacher authorizes us to love our enemies."[70]

Goldwater argued that "the truth of the matter is that the country cannot spare the number of graduate nurses that the army requires, nor can the training schools produce new graduates in sufficient numbers to satisfy the needs of both the military and the civilian population." Instead, he proposed

> the training of a large number of non-professional, voluntary war nursing aids, enlisted for the period of the war only, and composed of a class which will not take up nursing professionally under any circumstances, but which is willing to give gratuitous hospital service during the emergency.[71]

"We Do Not Know Classes in Nursing"

Goldwater thus explicitly raised the class issue: "The women I have in mind belong wholly or almost wholly to the leisure class. . . . When the war is over, the nursing aids will melt away into private life, leaving the nursing field in the hands of professional nurses."[72] Professional nursing leaders viewed the delicate issue of class distinctions with some ambivalence. Wealthy women had been their allies in many earlier battles, but having achieved a level of political sophistication that permitted it, professional nursing leaders increasingly sought to set themselves apart as a special group. Nutting revealed this ambivalence in her response, pointing out that such women would not necessarily "melt away" as predicted; "in England [they] are giving a good deal of trouble as they come back from France. They want to get registration [as nurses] not on the basis of study and training but because of their war experience. . . . They have the advantage of belonging to the 'leisure class' and frequently have title and wealth and position." However, Nutting added quickly, "We do not know classes in nursing; at least I hope we do not."[73] The prospect of a large number of untrained but influential women competing against trained nurses was precisely what nursing educators wanted to avert. Nutting made a coolly pointed rejoinder to Goldwater's proposal:

> There are two or three little points in Dr. Goldwater's very interesting discussion which I perhaps did not fully understand. I understood him to say that it was rather absurd to make the matter of housing student nurses determine the question of increasing the number of students, unless you increased, at the same time, the number of hospital beds. Surely Dr. Goldwater knows that in the State of New York there is, so far as we know, but one hospital that has established an eight hour day, and that hospitals can safely add to the number of nurses in their schools for some time yet, with the existing number of hospital beds, until the hours for students are made to conform to modern standards in the working world. Surely Dr. Goldwater knows that there are hospitals in New York City where the clinical facilities are excellent, and ample, but where it has been impossible to get reasonable hours for student nurses. . . . It has not seemed possible in certain hospitals to get anybody among large boards of wealthy trustees willing to take enough interest in their schools of nursing to provide sufficient accommodations to bring the hours of student nurses down to eight hours a day.[74]

The battle lines were being drawn. Goldwater had actually argued that increasing the number of pupil nurses would require increasing the number of hospital beds, since otherwise, presumably, the pupils would not be caring for enough patients to make their training experience adequate. Nutting neatly skewered this argument with her clear reference to Goldwater's own Mt. Sinai Hospital, where it was not until 1930 that pupil nurses obtained a forty-hour week, and not until 1950 that graduate nurses achieved the same.[75] One cannot but suspect that she viewed Goldwater as a doubtful friend of professional nursing, despite his rhetoric to the contrary.

"A Reasonable, Sensible Woman"

The next morning Delano addressed the group on "The Red Cross Aid Versus the Short-Term Course." She reminded the group that the aides had previously been authorized for the base hospital units, and asserted, "I hold no brief for nurses' aids as such, but I do hold a brief for your obligations and giving your word and then standing by it. For I am absolutely in sympathy with any plan that will help meet the needs of the country today."[76] For the Red Cross, she emphasized, "it is not at all a question for us of one thing as against the other. We are willing to help in any way we can."[77] But, she continued earnestly,

> I do feel that there is a place in the small hospital for hands and for feet more or less trained. I do feel that if I had a man in the service—and I regret that I have

none—but if I had a man in the service I should far rather that a reasonable, sensible woman would give him a drink of water when he was crying for it than that no one else should be there to give it to him.[78]

An urgency borne of the knowledge she held of the seriousness of the situation, based no doubt in part on the letters she received from nurses about conditions overseas, colored her speech:

> I think that it has somehow not come to us that this country is actually at war, and that if we do not win the war it will not make very much difference whether we have any training schools or not. If we do not win this war I do not care whether any of us are here a year from now . . . we have fought and we have bled and almost died for our nursing standards, and I do not believe that there is a nurse that has ever worked with me . . . that does not believe I would safeguard those to the last ditch, unless I felt that there was something more important, even, than our training school standards.
>
> Now what I want today is for the nurses of this country to forget everything except the importance of the need at this time.[79]

Delano asserted that the Red Cross was ready to carry out whatever decision was reached, but argued passionately, her white hair contrasting dramatically with the dark hollows under her eyes, that

> the only point that I think important and I will make is that we are not fair to the women of this country if we say absolutely, after five years of building up a service for them, and they are not yet accepted today, if we say, "We will have none of you." I think we have prejudiced our profession in the minds of the public by this attitude more than anything that has ever happened.[80]

Delano, who had spent long months working closely at the Red Cross with volunteer "leisure class" women, believed in nursing standards. But her compassion for the laywomen's position and her sense of the urgency of the situation were paramount. If need existed, Delano wanted to meet it, even if it meant the temporary sacrifice of dearly held professional goals. Dedicated laywomen could surely help in some way, even if it were merely by giving a wounded man a drink of water. "There are not such great social differences or differences of wealth," she concluded. "We would rather believe that at heart we are first, last and all the time women."[81]

The Army School Proposal

If Delano was the kind of leader one wants by one's side for the maternal support and moral inspiration she embodied, Goodrich was the kind of aggressive, tough leader one does not want as an adversary—a sort of savvy street fighter on a professional level. "Small but . . . impressive, wiry and forceful, with flashing eyes and a deep voice that carried to the farthest corner," Annie Goodrich followed Delano, as she had so many times in other circumstances.[82] At the podium, Goodrich gave a carefully constructed, short, and logical presentation, a marked contrast to Delano's persuasive use of personal feelings and specific anecdotal examples. She spoke first of how she had learned of the aide plan, making it explicit that Delano had known and assented to its implementation without consulting nursing leaders. "It was my opinion then," she asserted firmly, "and this opinion has not changed, that no step could be taken which would more greatly deflect young women from entering schools of nursing."[83]

Instead, the plan for the army school of nursing had been developed, over a series of meetings that, Goodrich was careful to note, Delano had attended. The proposed plan was for a three-year diploma course, during which the students would be serving in various base hospitals and receiving an allowance. "It is difficult to conceive," she added, "that anyone should not see the desirability of the method of using the aid as a student through the proposed school," and she argued that it would be an "injustice" to patients and to young women not to do so.[84]

Lively discussion followed. Nutting, of course, supported the army school plan. Obviously aware of Delano's loyal following and powers of persuasion, Nutting began by offering lavish praise for her work, then led the discussion smoothly toward the abstract and general and away from the specific:

> Miss Delano and I do not agree upon every point, but I always feel something go as soon as she begins with what she says, and I am carried along with her. Then I find myself asking a few little questions . . . volunteer nurses were created, to begin with, at a time when we had no professional body. . . . Miss Delano reminds us of our obligation. We should not forget the pledges that we have made . . . but when she asks us not to change our point of view, then I cannot agree with her. And what sanction do we have? We elected the president, a few years ago, on what ground? That he would keep us out of war; but he has changed his point of view. . . . I believe that as long as we live in a living, growing world, and circumstances change and conditions change, we must change our point of view. What are we in war for? Because a nation with whom we are at war cannot change her point of view.[85]

Emphasizing that she had "no hostility toward aids, I do not think the heavens would fall if we had 5,000 of them or 10,000 of them in the country. . . . I like many of the aids," Nutting asked the group to consider whether the aide plan was really "the best that we can do with our present knowledge and the present state of affairs."[86]

A Miss Burns spoke up, responding that, in the army,

> we accept everything that is available. The women of America who have given their sons, their husbands, their property, are willing to serve as privates now under officers as nurses, four privates to one nurse. . . . Are you going to turn down the private? . . . We have no moral, ethical or spiritual right to say, "you shall not serve as privates in the care of our men."[87]

But this traditionalist voice was in the minority. Further discussion followed, with Goodrich again pointing out that Delano had helped to develop the army school plan. Delano rose again, perhaps a bit defensively: "I never opposed the idea of a school for nurses," she emphasized. "I have cooperated with it. I was on the committee sitting while Miss Goodrich planned it out, and am entirely in sympathy with the idea." But, she added,

> I question whether it would meet the whole need and I question very seriously whether by approving of this plan, we would not absolutely eliminate all possibility of aids for service, even though we find the training school does not meet the needs and does not satisfy the women longing for service. . . . I feel very strongly that in adopting this plan we must not adopt it as an absolute substitute for the plan to which we are already pledged.[88]

The motion to establish an army school of nursing was carried on a voice vote. Whether Delano's qualification was accepted remains ambiguous, but, later in the meeting, Nutting managed to pass a resolution appointing a new committee, "very carefully considered," to study the question of training "attendants." "I think," Nutting emphasized, "we should make a careful study rather than take any hasty action."[89]

Steering "Between the Breakers"

Delano must be viewed as the loser in this struggle, along with the volunteer women whose position she had championed. "For the first time," wrote Sarah Pickett, "the rank and file of nurses had not followed her."[90] Delano returned to Red Cross Headquarters and promptly embarked on a massive recruitment drive to obtain nurses for the army. In February 1918, the surgeon general of the army had called for fifty thousand graduate and student nurses to be available by January 1919, a need which no doubt had added to Delano's sense of the desperateness of the situation. In a letter dated 25 March 1918, Delano had reported a need for 20,789 more nurses between March 1918 and January 1919; in 1917, enrollment had averaged only 817 per month.[91] The recruitment drive was carried out through the local divisions and chapters, and it was phenomenally successful. During the five months from July to December 1918, 11,118 nurses were enrolled.[92]

After another delay, during which the army general staff initially rejected the school plan, Goodrich and her allies brought pressure to bear. The school plan was finally approved 25 May 1918. Annie Goodrich was named dean, a development that is said to have greatly amused Isabel Stewart, since Goodrich was a confirmed pacifist.[93] But Goldwater had not given up. At the 27 May 1918 meeting of the Committee on Nursing, General Medical Board, Goldwater still maintained that the army school plan was "a national blunder," but the remaining members of the committee reiterated their view that aide training "constitutes an undesirable method of meeting the problems of either civilian or military nursing."[94] In June, at the meeting of the American Hospital Association, Goldwater continued to rail against the army school plan.[95] Goodrich wrote to Nutting on 28 July:

> We shall have no trouble whatever in meeting the nursing needs if people will stop saying that we have got to come to aids. I think Dr. Goldwater is mean enough to keep this up just because it is the best way to deflect students and he wants to injure the school. Col. Smith thinks it is because he wants to keep himself in the public eye.[96]

Delano, torn between her loyalty to professional nursing, her loyalty to the Red Cross, and her loyalty to the women volunteers whose preparation she had shepherded through years of effort, wrote to Sophia Palmer on 8 June 1918: "I am kept busy trying to steer my craft between the breakers, believing as I do that both sides are right and both sides are wrong. With your understanding mind, you will know what I mean."[97]

Having attained their goal of an army school, Nutting and Goodrich apparently looked with more tolerance on the question of aides, for at a meeting of the Committee on Nursing, Council of National Defense held in September, unanimous approval was given to a motion by Goldwater calling for the training of hospital assistants for service in civil, Red Cross, or military hospitals.[98] Even so, Goldwater continued on the warpath; an editorial in the September issue of *The Modern Hospital,* entitled "Once more the Army nursing question," argued for aide courses to prepare units similar to the aide divisions in use in England.[99] The next month, he pushed through adoption of a resolution by the Hospital Conference of New York City, which urged preparation of an aide training program by the surgeon general's office, in conjunction with the American Hospital Association, as a substitute for a "makeshift proposal" involving the surgeon general and the army nursing school.[100] But despite all Goldwater's efforts to sabotage it, the "Department of Nursing" column in the same issue trumpeted that "the army school has triumphantly solved the problem of nursing in our many cantonment hospitals."[101]

Throughout the autumn, Delano and her associates worked frenziedly to meet the needs of the military as well as the civilian population, which was in the throes of an influenza epidemic that would eventually kill 400,000 people in the United States.[102] Clara Noyes, speaking of working with Delano during this trying time, said later,

> many times when we reached the end of a weary day's work and the pressure seemed almost more than human power could stand I have heard her say, when asked if she were tired, "Well, I suppose it is no harder for us to die at our desks than for the boys to die in the trenches."[103]

Postscript

But Delano was not to die at her desk. The armistice was signed in November 1918, and in December she took the time to write to her old friend Sylveen Nye before sailing to France for an inspection tour of Red Cross facilities. "Just as soon as this war is over, you and I start out 'Veenie' and we'll see the Earth," she wrote. "It makes no difference, North, East, or South; we shall buy no return ticket."[104] She was not to see her friend again. Delano died in France of a mastoid infection while on her tour.[105]

Goodrich launched the army school, which operated until 1932 when it closed due to economic constraints.[106] In 1923 she went on to become the dean of the Yale University School of Nursing, living to see to fruition her early dreams for college-prepared nurses. Goldwater became a sought-after consultant on hospitals, who quoted Florence Nightingale in essays on hospital organization.[107] The aide question, however, as evidenced by the American Medical Association's late and little-lamented proposal for Registered Care Technicians to solve a nursing shortage, has never been put to rest.

Conclusion

Delano, caught "on the fence" in this conflict, is a transitional figure in whom we find traces of both the older, nineteenth-century ideals of nursing as a calling, as women's work, as service or duty, and the professionalist forces that in the twentieth century elevated professional expertise and technical skill over personal moral commitment. But the traditionalist view was predominant in Delano. "Self has been crucified," she wrote in her last report to the *American Journal of Nursing,* "and in its place has arisen service."[108] Both Delano, drawn to nursing by a missionary's compassion for the suffering, and Goodrich, drawn to nursing by her determined desire to improve her lot in life, personify conflicting forces still firmly embedded in an occupation that seeks to combine altruistic service with the sometimes contradictory exclusivity and autonomy of professionalism.[109] Was Delano a saint or a sellout? Our answer will depend on the balance we strike between the rational and the intuitive; between nursing as theory and nursing as practice; between nursing as noun and nursing as verb; between nursing as science and nursing as art.[110]

Ruth E. Malone, RN, MS
Doctoral Student
School of Nursing
University of California, San Francisco

3906 Midvale Avenue
Oakland, Calif. 94602
Phone: (510) 531-3136

Acknowledgments

Support for work on this manuscript was provided by a University of California Regents Fellowship. The author gratefully acknowledges the assistance of David M. Weinberg, Curator, Center for the Study of the History of Nursing; Marilyn Flood, RN, PhD, Dean for Academic Affairs, School of Nursing, UCSF; Jackie Berry, American Red Cross Archives; and the very helpful comments of Joan Lynaugh, RN, PhD, and two anonymous reviewers. And special thanks to my mother, Orva Bess Malone, my father, W. W. Malone, and my husband, Terry Sayre, without whose steadfast encouragement this work would not have been possible.

Notes

1. Minnie Goodnow, *Outlines of Nursing History* (Philadelphia, Pa.: W. B. Saunders, 1937), 18.

2. Mary A. Clark, *Memories of Jane A. Delano* (New York: Lakeside Publishing Company, 1934), 3.

3. Mary M. Roberts, *American Nursing: History and Interpretation* (New York: Macmillan, 1954), 76. Also see "Honor Roll," *American Journal of Nursing* 19, no. 8 (May 1919): 650 (hereafter cited as *AJN*), which observes that Delano "was without doubt the most widely known, personally, throughout the country, of any of our leading nurses."

4. "Jane A. Delano Memorial Services," *AJN* 11, no. 9 (June 1919): 657–60. Also see "Miss Delano's Grave," *AJN* 19, no. 12 (September 1919): 912–15; "Memorial to Miss Delano," *AJN* 20, no. 9 (June 1920): 716; "Miss Delano's Body Laid to Rest in Arlington," *AJN* 21, no. 1 (October 1920): 38; Julia C. Stimson, "Miss Delano, The Great Nurse, Laid to Rest in Arlington," *AJN* 21, no. 1 (October 1920): 96–97; "American Nurses Honored in Memory of the Late Jane A. Delano," *AJN* 21, no. 4 (September 1921): 246; and "Memorial to Jane A. Delano," *AJN* 22, no. 1 (November 1921): 108.

5. Lavinia L. Dock et al., eds., *History of American Red Cross Nursing* (New York: Macmillan, 1922), 962.

6. Portia B. Kernodle, *The Red Cross Nurse in Action, 1882–1948* (New York: Harper and Bros., 1949), 135.

7. Jerome Burne, *Chronicle of the World* (Paris and London: Ecam Publications, 1989), 1072.

8. Goodnow, 439.

9. *Proceedings, Twenty-fourth Annual Convention, National League for Nursing Education* (Cleveland, 1918), 162 (hereafter cited as *Proceedings, NLNE24*).

10. Isabel A. Hampton, "Educational Standards for Nurses," in *Nursing of the Sick*, ed. Isabel A. Hampton (International Congress of Charities, Correction, and Philanthropy, Chicago, 3rd Section, 1893; reprint, New York: McGraw-Hill, 1949), 5.

11. Dock et al., 958.

12. Clark, 8, 12. J. R. Coddington, in 1912, wrote about the qualities desired in a nursing superintendent:

> She should be selected with unusual consideration and caution. If the nurses are to look up to her as their guide and counselor, as they should, she must be first of all, a true gentlewoman, of broad education, with the necessary nurses' training, and will power sufficient to govern herself and others; also tact and ability. She must be a teacher and a disciplinarian, able to govern justly and rightly. . . . No position in life gives a woman the opportunity to impress herself on the lives of so many young women and to such a degree. . . . She stands, in my mind, next to a mother in her opportunities, and in one respect with her they are greater, for so many more come under her care and influence.

J. R. Coddington, "Hospital Management, Especially the Division of Responsibility and Labor," *Transactions, American Hospital Association,* Fourteenth Annual Conference (1912), 14:140–41.

13. Dorothy Giles, *A Candle in Her Hand: A Story of the Nursing Schools of Bellevue Hospital* (New York: G. P. Putnam's Sons, 1949), 178.

14. Mary E. Gladwin, *The Red Cross and Jane Arminda Delano* (Philadelphia: W. B. Saunders, 1931), 36.

15. Clark, 6.

16. Dock et al., 1361.

17. Jane A. Delano and Isabel I. McIsaac, *American Red Cross Textbook on Elementary Hygiene and Home Care of the Sick* (Philadelphia, Pa.: P. Blakiston's Sons, 1914), xv.

18. Dock et al., 1370.

19. Ibid., 234.

20. Ibid., 207–8.

21. Ibid., 209.

22. Anonymous, *Mademoiselle Miss: Letters From an American Girl Serving With The Rank of Lieutenant in a French Army Hospital at the Front* (Boston, Mass.: W. A. Butterfield, 1916), 37–38. This same writer offers a description of what is required of a nurse at the front:

> To be ideally suited to the post she should combine a glacial calm with the unfailing gayety of springtime, and a sense of humor always; she should possess law and order and arrangement, the powers of construction and invention, a touch as light as a watchmaker's, and strength to carry a man alone on occasion; she should combine tremendous initiative with excessive caution, firmness with tenderness, authority with courtesy, fearlessness with awe, and she ought to be a psychologist, and deeply learned in the profession, and ready to read the riot-act when called for.

23. Dock et al.

24. Kernodle, 122–23.

25. See letter from S. S. Goldwater to A. S. Downing, 28 July 1917, arguing for aide courses. Archives, Department of Nursing Education, Division of Nursing Education, Teachers College, Columbia University (hereafter cited as DNE-TC).

26. Kernodle, 125–26. Kernodle also notes the stunning growth in Red Cross membership during the war years: In 1916 membership was 286,461; by 1918 it was 30,000,000.

27. Minutes, Committee on Nursing, Council of National Defense, 10 November 1917, DNE-TC.

28. Goldwater resigned from Nutting's committee 18 September 1918, noting that with the approval of the Army school, he felt confident there would be no further need for "constructive criticism." S. S. Goldwater to Dr. Franklin H. Martin, 18 September 1918, DNE-TC.

29. Susan M. Reverby, *Ordered to Care: The Dilemma of American Nursing, 1850–1945* (New York: Cambridge University Press, 1989). Reverby has noted that

institutional connections were a key source of the network of "elite" nurses who constituted most of the nursing leadership: "Of ninety women identified as leaders in nursing between 1873 and 1945, nearly fifty percent (forty-four) trained in only six major large nursing schools located in teaching hospitals: Johns Hopkins, Bellevue, New York Hospital, Boston City, Massachusetts General, and Connecticut Training School-Yale New Haven" (124).

30. Historians have noted the two-track system that existed in the larger nursing schools. While the majority of graduates went to private duty nursing in the homes of middle- or upper-class families, a very small group were selected to be superintendents in hospital schools. These women tended to have come from better social backgrounds, and their selection meant more status and more potential for advancement. See Nancy Tomes, "'Little World of Our Own': The Pennsylvania Hospital Training School for Nurses, 1895–1907," in *Women and Health in America,* ed. Judith W. Leavitt (Madison: University of Wisconsin, 1984), 467–81; C. E. Rosenberg, *In the Care of Strangers* (New York: Basic Books, 1987), 225.

31. However, their exclusivity left them open to criticism. Dr. Anita Newcomb McGee, a physician who was generally supportive of nurses, remarked in 1900 that the Associated Alumnae, "though theoretically a society of nurses, has up to the present been practically an aristocracy of schools." Anita Newcomb McGee, "The Standard of Trained Nursing in America," *Trained Nurse and Hospital Review* 25, no. 2 (August 1900): 94 (hereafter cited as *TN*). Dr. McGee, who directed army nursing during the Spanish-American War, later incurred the ire of organized professional nurses by resisting their efforts to place army nurses under the direct authority of a nurse. See Susan Armeny, "Organized Nurses, Women Philanthropists, and the Intellectual Bases for Cooperation Among Women, 1898–1920," in *Nursing History: New Perspectives, New Possibilities,* ed. Ellen C. Lagemann (New York: Teachers College Press, 1983), 13–45.

32. In Dock et al., 965.

33. Anna H. Erdmann, "Miss Delano Through the Eyes of a Lifelong Friend, Sylveen Nye," *TN* 106 (April 1941): 280–81.

34. Harriet B. Koch, *Militant Angel* (New York: Macmillan, 1951), 14. This biography was written, with her consultation, while Goodrich was still alive.

35. Esther A. Werminghaus, *Annie W. Goodrich: Her Journey to Yale* (New York: MacMillan, 1950), 8.

36. Edna Yost, *American Women of Nursing* (Philadelphia, Pa.: Lippincott, 1947), 45.

37. Quoted in T. E. Christy, "Portrait of a Leader: Annie Warburton Goodrich," in *Pages From Nursing History* (New York: American Journal of Nursing Company, 1984), 76–80.

38. Dock et al., 540–58, chronicle these events. Sarah Pickett, author of the chapter "The European War," in which these events are discussed, expresses doubt that "elements of personal interest were guiding factors on either side of the case" (558). But subsequent events raise this possibility.

39. Ibid., 553.

40. Ibid., 554.

41. Ibid., 554–55.

42. Ibid., 555–56.

43. Ibid., 556–57.

44. Ibid., 557.

45. Barbara Melosh, *The Physician's Hand* (Philadelphia, Pa.: Temple University Press, 1982), 22.

46. Editorial comment, *TN* 25, no. 3 (September 1900): 198.

47. *Proceedings, NLNE24,* 169.

48. Georgia M. Nevins, "As Known By Her Friends," *AJN* 19, no. 9 (June 1919): 700.

49. Delano left an estate valued at more than half a million dollars at her death in 1919. See "The Will of Jane A. Delano," *AJN* 19, no. 10 (July 1919): 746–47.

50. Erdmann, 280.

51. Armeny, 13–45.

52. Mary A. Messner, "Is Nursing A Profession?" *AJN* 15, no. 2 (November 1914): 122–23.

53. William C. Gorgas to Secretary of War, 30 January 1918, Mary Adelaide Nutting Papers, History of Nursing Archives, Teachers College, Columbia University (hereafter cited as MAN Papers).

54. Telegram, Ella P. Crandall to M. Adelaide Nutting, 30 January 1918; Winford H. Smith to M. Adelaide Nutting, 15 February 1918, MAN Papers.

55. Dock et al.

56. Annie Goodrich to M. Adelaide Nutting, undated letter, MAN Papers.

57. Telegram and letter, M. Adelaide Nutting to Jane A. Delano, 20 February 1918, MAN Papers.

58. M. Adelaide Nutting to Annie Goodrich, 21 February 1918, MAN Papers.

59. Handwritten letter, Annie Goodrich to M. Adelaide Nutting, 20 February 1918, MAN Papers. Delano, however, was perhaps more aware of the urgency of the situation. In a letter to Mrs. John Sinclair, dated 25 March 1918, she noted that there were 65,084 graduate nurses in the country and forecasted a need of 20,789 between March 1918 and January 1919 (DNE-TC).

60. Handwritten letter, Annie Goodrich to M. Adelaide Nutting, 26 February 1918, MAN Papers.

61. Handwritten letter, Annie Goodrich to M. Adelaide Nutting, 29 March 1918, MAN Papers.

62. M. Adelaide Nutting to Annie Goodrich, 23 December 1918, MAN Papers.

63. Editorial, "The Nursing Profession and the National Crisis," *The Modern Hospital* 10, no. 4 (April 1918): 275–76 (hereafter cited as *MH*).

64. This sort of perspective on the shortage of nurses remains in evidence today. For a current example, see Joan Lynaugh, "Riding the Yo-Yo: The Worth and Work of Nursing in the Twentieth Century," *Transactions and Studies of the College of Physicians of Philadelphia* 11 (September 1989): 201–17.

65. Charles B. Grimshaw, "The Nursing Profession and The Two-Year Training Course," *MH* 10, no. 5 (May 1918): 374–75.

66. J. E. Cutler, "How the Public and the Nursing Profession are Combining

to Supply Nursing Needs During and After the War: Approach from the Standpoint of the Educator Looking Toward the Future," *Proceedings, NLNE24*, 122–23.

67. M. Adelaide Nutting, "How the Nursing Profession is Trying to Meet the Problems Arising Out of the War," *Proceedings, NLNE24*, 130.

68. Hospitals had just come through a period characterized by economic difficulty, and their administrators feared more of the same. See David Rosner, "Business At the Bedside: Health Care in Brooklyn, 1890–1915," in *Health Care in America: Essays in Social History,* ed. Susan Reverby and David Rosner (Philadelphia, Pa.: Temple University Press, 1979), 117–31. Also see S. S. Goldwater, "War-Time Savings," *MH* 10, no. 5 (May 1918): 349–50; "War Service Committee Conference," *MH* 11, no. 1 (July 1918): 35–42.

69. For a biographical introduction to Goldwater's life and a collection of his essays, see S. S. Goldwater, *On Hospitals* (New York: Macmillan, 1947).

70. *Proceedings, NLNE24*, 131–32.

71. S. S. Goldwater, "The Nursing Crisis: Efforts to Satisfy the Nursing Requirements of the War, A Way Out of the Difficulty," *Proceedings, NLNE24*, 138.

72. Ibid., 139.

73. Ibid., 141.

74. Ibid., 140. For a more glowing report on the conditions for pupil nurses at Mt. Sinai Hospital at the time, see Margaret J. Robinson, "Little Journeys to Places and People Worth Knowing," *MH* 11, no. 6 (December 1918): 454–57. Also see Joseph Hirsh and Beka Doherty, *The First Hundred Years of the Mt. Sinai Hospital of New York* (New York: Random House, 1952).

75. Personal communication, 29 May 1992, from Archivist, Mt. Sinai Hospital, New York City.

76. Jane A. Delano, "Red Cross Aid Versus the Short-Term Course," *Proceedings, NLNE24*, 164.

77. Ibid., 165.

78. Ibid., 166.

79. Ibid., 166.

80. Ibid., 169.

81. Ibid., 171.

82. According to Kernodle, 137.

83. Annie W. Goodrich, "The Plan for the Army School of Nursing," *Proceedings, NLNE24*, 172.

84. Ibid., 174.

85. *Proceedings, NLNE24*, 183–84.

86. Ibid., 184.

87. Ibid., 185.

88. Ibid., 190.

89. Ibid., 269.

90. Dock et al., 964.

91. Jane A. Delano to Mrs. John Sinclair, 25 March 1918, DNE-TC.

92. Jane A. Delano, Tenth Annual Report of the Nursing Service, American Red Cross, June 30, 1917–July 1, 1918, No. 140.18 Nursing Service Reports, cited in

G. R. Gaeddert, *The History of the American National Red Cross, Vol. IV* (Washington, D.C.: American National Red Cross, 1950), 264–65.

93. Christy, 78.

94. Committee on Nursing, Council of National Defense, General Medical Board, 27 May 1918, DNE-TC.

95. William H. Walsh, "War Service Committee Conference," reported in *MH* 11, no. 1 (July 1918): 35–42. Also see S. S. Goldwater, "The Nursing Crisis: Insufficiency of Supply of Graduate Nurses to Meet War Needs—No Prospect of Adequate Increase—Dangers of Breaking Down Standards—Training of Nursing Aids the Solution," *MH* 10, no. 6 (June 1918).

96. Annie Goodrich to M. Adelaide Nutting, 28 July 1918, MAN Papers. Another letter from Goodrich to Nutting, of unknown date, complains that Goldwater's "behavior has been so dastardly . . . I feel sick . . . of struggling with him" (MAN Papers).

97. Cited in Dock et al., 963. Delano did support the army school, however. See Jane A. Delano, "The Nursing Program of the American Red Cross," *MH* 11, no. 4 (October 1918): 336–38, where she notes: "Never before in the history of nursing has it been attempted to man large hospitals varying in size from several hundred to several thousand beds with a graduate service of nurses. Nor is it believed that even in time of war this is the best form of hospital administration. It is hoped that the Army School of Nursing will supply the greatly needed supplementary service."

98. Dock et al. This program, however, was planned for women not meeting the requirements of the army school, such as those who were married and single women thirty-five to forty-five years old. See Annie Goodrich, "The Nursing Program of the Army," *MH* 11, no. 5 (November 1918): 410–13.

99. "Once More the Army Nursing Question," editorial, *MH* 11, no. 3 (September 1918): 189–90. As late as October 1918, Goldwater was still arguing for volunteer aides. See "Report of the War Service Committee," *MH* 11, no. 4 (October 1918): 332–34. Goldwater chaired this committee.

100. "The Civil Hospitals and the Army Nursing School," *MH* 11, no. 4 (October 1918): 290. In the same issue, an article by M. Adelaide Nutting, "The Relation of the War Program to Nursing in Civil Hospitals," notes "a decided reaction going on against short superficial courses of training," 341.

101. Mabelle S. Welsh, "The Standard Curriculum for Schools of Nursing," *MH* 11, no. 4 (October 1918): 303.

102. Clara D. Noyes, "The Red Cross Nursing Service at Home and Abroad," in *Proceedings, Twenty-Fifth Annual Convention, National League for Nursing Education* (Chicago: NLNE, June 1919), 135–45. For more on the influenza epidemic of 1918, see Jane A. Delano, "Meeting the Spanish Influenza Situation," *AJN* 19, no. 2 (November 1918): 108–11; Editorial, "The Epidemic of Influenza," *AJN* 19, no. 2 (November 1918): 83–85; Jane A. Delano, "Greater Love Hath No Man," *AJN* 19, no. 3 (December 1918): 185–88; American National Red Cross, *The Mobilisation of the American National Red Cross During the Influenza Pandemic, 1918–1919* (Washington, D.C.: American Red Cross, 1920); and Gaeddert, *History of the American National Red Cross, Vol. IV*.

103. Noyes, 145.

104. Erdmann, 281.

105. For details of her death, see Edna L. Foley, "Last Honors," *AJN* 19, no. 9 (June 1919): 688–95. Delano herself summarized the work of the war years in a piece printed after she had sailed for France. See Jane A. Delano, "How American Nurses Helped Win The War," *MH* 12, no. 1 (January 1919): 7–9.

106. Goodnow, 1937. Annie Goodrich, to her credit, spoke warmly of Delano at the graduation of the first class from the army school of nursing in 1921. Her address, and a tribute to Delano, are reprinted in Annie W. Goodrich, *The Social and Ethical Significance of Nursing* (New York: Macmillan, 1932).

107. S. S. Goldwater, *On Hospitals* (New York: Macmillan, 1947).

108. Delano, "Greater Love Hath No Man," 185.

109. Nancy Tomes, in a cogent analysis of the 1918 crisis, points out that professional nurses elevated their social worth at the expense of their lay volunteer sisters, and in the process devalued volunteerism and caring itself. What was a gain for professional nurses, as we have seen, may after all have been a loss for women as a whole. See Nancy Tomes, "A Collision of Nursing's Two Worlds: Volunteer and Professional Nurses in World War I" (Paper given at the Fifth Berkshire Conference on the History of Women, Vassar College, Poughkeepsie, N.Y., 18 June 1981). Cited with permission of the author.

110. For further perspectives on the historical tension between professionalism and caring, see Ellen D. Baer, "Of Exclusion and Divided Houses," *Nursing Research* 39, no. 5 (September/October 1990): 318–19; Patricia O'Brien, "'All A Woman's Life Can Bring': The Domestic Roots of Nursing in Philadelphia, 1830–1885," *Nursing Research* 36, no. 1 (January/February 1987): 12–17; Reverby, *Ordered to Care;* Melosh, *The Physician's Hand.* A more contemporary discussion of this tension may be found in Patricia Benner and Judith Wrubel, *The Primacy of Caring: Stress and Coping in Health and Illness* (Menlo Park, Calif.: Addison-Wesley, 1989), 365–88.

"Of Logical Necessity . . . They Hang Together": Nursing and the Woman's Movement, 1901–1912

Sandra Lewenson
College of Nursing
State University of New York
Health Science Center at Brooklyn

Introduction

With the approval of the executive boards of the American Society of Superintendents of Training Schools for Nurses (hereafter the Superintendents' Society) and the Nurses' Associated Alumnae of the United States and Canada (hereafter the Associated Alumnae), a "marriage" of convenience took place in 1901 between America's two nursing organizations, resulting in the American Federation of Nurses (hereafter the Federation). This alliance permitted America's two professional associations to formally participate in the activities of the woman's movement through membership in the National Council of Women (NCW) of the United States and the International Council of Women (ICW). Membership in the NCW granted the newly organized Federation the "privileges of membership in the great [international] congresses of women meeting every five years."[1] The Federation, like other women's groups at that time, had to enter the National Council of Women first in order to become part of the ICW. Although its membership in the NCW lasted until 1905, the Federation continued to represent American organized nursing in the ICW and later in the International Council of Nurses (ICN) until 1912.

One of the driving forces behind this union came from nursing leader and staunch suffragist Lavinia Dock (1858–1956), who saw the important role nurses could play in the unfolding national and international struggle for women's rights. Dock convincingly argued that organized nursing should enter the international movement of women that collectively advo-

Nursing History Review 2 (1994): 99–117.

ORGANIZATIONAL TIMELINE

1848	Woman's Rights Convention in Seneca Falls held
1888	International Council of Women (ICW) established
1888	National Council of Women (NCW) established
1893	American Society of Superintendents of Training Schools for Nurses (Superintendents' Society) established
1893	Chicago Columbian Exposition held
1893	ICW First Quinquennial in Chicago held
1894	Matron's Council of Great Britain and Ireland established
1896	Nurses' Associated Alumnae of the United States and Canada (Associated Alumnae) established
1899	International Council of Nurses (ICN) established
1899	ICW Quinquennial in London
1901	American Federation of Nurses (Federation) established
1901	ICN meets at the Pan American Exposition in Buffalo
1905	Federation withdraws from the NCW and joins the ICN
1908	National Association of Colored Graduate Nurses (NACGN) established
1909	ICN meets in London
1911	Associated Alumnae becomes the American Nurses' Association (ANA)
1912	National Organization of Public Health Nursing (NOPHN) established
1912	Superintendents' Society renamed the National League of Nursing Education
1912	ANA represents American nursing at the ICN in Cologne, Germany

cated and argued for the personal and professional rights of women. This article explores the reasons why America's two national nursing organizations' formed the Federation, chronicles the Federation's eleven-year history, and argues that through this affiliation, organized nursing engaged in the political activities of the woman's movement and subsequently supported the national and international drive for woman suffrage.[2]

Professional Nursing Organizations

The two national professional organizations originally formed to address problems inherent in the apprenticeship system of education in the hospital training schools, and the conditions of nursing practice. The Superintendents' Society limited its membership to the superintendents of nurse training schools and sought control and advancement of nurses' education. The Associated Alumnae promoted and supported trained nurses working in all other nursing positions. Sophia Palmer (1853–1920), Dock's colleague and the first editor of the *American Journal of Nursing* (*AJN*), considered organization to be the "power of the day."[3] She edited the journal as a forum within which nurses could address their professional concerns. Like other nursing leaders, Palmer felt that inconsistent nursing curriculums, nursing students' long hours of service to the hospital, too few years spent in training, lack of state nursing registration laws, unregulated nursing directories, and exploitation of nursing could only be addressed through nursing organizations. Having recognized that organization meant power to change, American nurses willingly engaged in the activities of the international movement of women to gain equal political and social status for women.

The American Federation of Nurses

Mary Thornton, an 1890 graduate of the New York Post-Graduate Medical School and Hospital and secretary of its alumnae association, urged the nursing class of 1901 to join the school's alumnae association, thus becoming eligible to attend the International Council of Nurses Congress that would be held in Buffalo, New York, on 6 September 1901. "There, too," Thornton continued, "we shall have for the first time representation in the National Council of Women. . . . Surely you will want to take part in this history-making epoch of your profession."[4] Thornton was not alone in her sentiments; many others in nursing felt similar enthusiasm for organization and affiliation among nurses and women. By 1901, women, politically frustrated because they lacked the franchise, established a network of organizations to rectify the social ills of society. Lavinia Dock stood among those who advocated social reform and the formation of women's associations. Dock committed her time and expertise to the founding of the first two national nursing organizations in the United States: the Superintendents' Society in 1893 and Associated Alumnae in 1896. Once established, Dock pursued an alliance of these two professional groups with other national and international women's groups. She persistently argued her position among colleagues, explaining that the rights of trained nurses were intricately woven with the rights of women. Dock believed that women's political power depended on the strength achieved through associations among women and zealously advocated nursing's affiliation with other women's groups that formed at the beginning of the twentieth century. She used the *AJN,* first published in 1900, as a vehicle to inform nurses of international events that impinged on the professional development of nursing and on the political freedom of all women. Dock believed that the way to gain professional rights as nurses was to gain basic rights as women.

Dock's continued effort to unite the newly formed American nursing organizations with the ICW succeeded, and in 1901, without having to disrupt the distinct purpose of either the Superintendents' Society or the Associated Alumnae, the American Federation of Nurses formed. Between 1901 and 1912, the Federation provided the Superintendents' Society and the Associated Alumnae access into other women's groups and thus afforded trained nurses the opportunity to be part of what Mary Thornton described as a history-making epoch.

Reasons Why the Federation Formed

Only through an organization could individuals affiliate with the NCW, and only through the NCW could organizations join the ICW. Hence, the Superintendents' Society and the Associated Alumnae first had to enter the NCW in order to affiliate with the International Council of Women. After much debate about this eligibility problem, the two nursing organizations found it more economical and politically astute to join the NCW and the ICW as one representative professional group; they formed the American

Federation of Nurses in 1901 to do so. Dock explained that the idea for a Federation was recommended by the president of the NCW, May Wright Sewall, who had encouraged the two associations to affiliate without altering the goals of their respective groups. The main purpose of the Federation was to prepare members to become "one representative body ready to unite in friendly relations with national societies in other countries."[5]

During these deliberations, Sewall explained in a letter to the Superintendents' Society why they should consider membership in the NCW and subsequently the ICW. The primary objective of the NCW, Sewall wrote, was to "promote the advancement of human society through the enlargement of the recognition of women in various industries and professions."[6] Thus, Sewall concluded, it seemed only natural that the Superintendents' Society "should be affiliated with other organizations in the Council."[7] In this way, she thought, nurses from many nations would be better served.[8]

The British president of the ICN, Ethel Fenwick, confirmed the importance of joining the NCW. Like Sewall, Fenwick wanted nurses to join the newly proposed ICN, but not at the expense of losing membership in the ICW; thus, Fenwick encouraged the respective national professional nursing groups to join their country's own NCW.[9]

After debating the issue, the superintendents decided to join the NCW at their seventh annual meeting in 1900. They supported entrance into the ICW as well as maintenance of a separate membership in the ICN. The superintendents wanted the newly formed Associated Alumnae to join the NCW with them but had to wait for them to agree. The Associated Alumnae in turn received an invitation to join the NCW from Fenwick. At meetings they discussed the reasons for joining and entertained the idea of affiliating with the Superintendents' Society to do so.[10] Members of the Associated Alumnae listened while their president, Isabel Hampton Robb, addressed them in May 1900 and again urged nurses to unite in "professional bonds" with nurses in other countries and to become identified with "woman's work" all over the world. In this way, Hampton Robb continued, nursing would gain "additional breadth and strength for our own more specialized efforts."[11]

Dock, as secretary of the Superintendents' Society and secretary of the ICN, advised that an affiliation between nursing's two professional organizations would enable the members of both groups to join the NCW. This, Dock argued, would bring American nurses closer to other women throughout the United States and abroad. Pragmatically, Dock explained that through a federation, the two organizations would share the expensive one-hundred dollar NCW membership fee as well as develop a strong political front.[12]

The association's membership frequently debated the issue of whether or not to join the NCW or just the ICN. When President Hampton Robb asked Dock if the Associated Alumnae could join the ICN without joining the NCW, Dock responded that it was "of logical necessity that they hang together."[13] Dock explained further, "We can only share in the quinquennial, where our International Council of Nurses will meet, by belonging to the National Council of our country."[14]

It was not clear why Dock said that membership in the ICN first required a membership in the NCW, since the ICN permitted individual memberships in 1901. This requirement changed in 1904 at the Berlin meeting, and membership could only be gained through an affiliating organization. Initially, in 1899, the Provisional Committee for the ICN allowed membership only through a national council like the ICW. However, the ICN could not enforce such a rule because few countries had national nursing associations. To stimulate "organization in other lands," then, the ICN encouraged individual membership, with the provision that once national nursing associations formed, membership would be open only to them.[15]

In spite of the confusion surrounding memberships in these international councils, nurses in the United States wanted to belong to this international woman's movement. At the third session of the 1900 Associated Alumnae's convention, nursing delegate Jessie Breeze read a resolution that called for the merger of the Associated Alumnae and the Superintendents' Society in order to apply for membership in the NCW and the ICW. In the motion, Breeze asked that two members from the Superintendents' Society and the Associated Alumnae, as well as two members-at-large, be appointed. Assured by Dock that the superintendents supported this union, the Associated Alumnae carried the proposed resolution.[16]

Women's Councils

By the dawn of the twentieth century, women had organized national and international councils to collectively argue for their rights as citizens. In March 1888 in Washington, D.C., the National Woman's Suffrage Association celebrated the fortieth anniversary of the Seneca Falls Woman's Rights Convention of 1848. Pioneer suffragists such as Susan B. Anthony (1820–

1906), Elizabeth Cady Stanton (1815–1902), Frances Willard (1839–1898), and May Wright Sewall (1844–1920) planned this event and invited women involved in "social, intellectual, moral, or civic reform."[17] Representatives from fifty-three national organizations, and forty-nine delegates from England, France, Denmark, Norway, Finland, India, Canada, and the United States came to Washington to celebrate and subsequently organize the ICW. Membership in the ICW was to consist of national councils from different countries representing the numerous women's organizations regardless of their political position on woman suffrage.[18]

The NCW of the United States, which had its origins at the meeting held in Washington, D.C., in 1888, became the means by which women in this country joined the ICW. Some of the women's groups that participated in the founding of this first national council included the National Woman's Christian Temperance Union, the National Woman's Relief Society, and the Young Woman's Mutual Improvement Association of the Church of Latter Day Saints. Over time, the council grew in numbers and encompassed most of the nation's women's associations, including the General Federation of Women's Clubs, Child Study Association of America, National Council of Jewish Women, and the National Association of Colored Women.

The NCW concerned itself with issues that confronted women's responsibilities in the home and in the country and protested "against persecution of any people."[19] Moreover, it promised to address the needs of people regardless of color, religion, or creed and promoted laws affirming the rights of women in the political, social, and economic realm. Since the council represented such a vast number of women's groups, the membership within the council reflected a wide range of women from different social, ethnic, and political backgrounds and ideologies. However, the social reformers of that era came from the educated middle- and upper-classes. Under the heading of social feminism, many of these women sought to improve social conditions in America for the urban poor, the immigrant labor force, and for women. Cities with a plethora of social ills offered many women a "large house" to sweep clean and reform. The social housekeeping activities of these organizations harnessed the energy of newly educated middle-class women who advocated advancing women's education, work, and rights while retaining the culture of women's separate sphere.[20]

The NCW served as a clearinghouse for information on the activities of the burgeoning number of women's organizations in the United States.

Describing itself as analogous to the "Industrial Machine," the NCW served as "the engine" for its member organizations—to "unite and concentrate scattered forces and amalgamate them into one."[21] In 1893, the same year as the founding of the Superintendents' Society, the NCW sponsored the first quinquennial meeting of the ICW at the Columbian Exposition in Chicago, from 15 to 22 May. Reported to be the "largest international gathering of women held up to that time," the international congress enabled the affiliating organizations to join with other "women's movements throughout the world."[22] One month later at the Chicago exposition, nursing leaders Lavinia Dock, Isabel Hampton Robb (1860–1910), and Sophia Palmer must have heard of the events of the Woman's Congress and seen the potential that affiliation with other women's organizations could have for nursing. These leaders, among others, wanted the nursing profession to be a part of the "engine" that would harness the power from a national and international association of women's groups, thus creating a broad-based alliance for the sought-after changes in nursing education and practice.[23]

International Council of Nurses

Ten years later, the International Council of Nurses (ICN), formed by the Matron's Council of Great Britain and Ireland (hereafter called the Matron's Council), met for the first time at the second International Council of Women's Quinquennial Meeting, held in London in 1899. Lavinia Dock had traveled with her sister Mira to attend the London Congress. Dock noted that the other American nurses who attended had found their way to the congress in a "hap-hazard" fashion, either because "they happened to be in England or because they were personally interested and curious to see what a great congress of women would be like."[24]

Once at that Congress, however, the American nurses had an opportunity to visit the Nursing Section, which had been placed on the program at the International Women's Congress at the insistence of English nursing organizer Ethel Gordon Fenwick (1857–1947). Being "something quite new in women's gatherings," the Nursing Section, Dock noted, had drawn little attention from nursing organizations in the United States, and hence they had had no official delegations present to represent them.[25]

While the ICW convened in London, trained nurses from America, Canada, Australia, Denmark, and Holland who attended the International

Women's Congress met at Fenwick's invitation. Fenwick and the Matron's Council had pioneered the initial meeting of nursing's international council, establishing it as one of the first professional international councils. The Matron's Council had been formed in 1894 by English superintendents who staunchly supported English nurses' drive for registration. Fenwick invited the ICW nursing delegates and the members of the Matron's Council to write the constitution for the new ICN. "Self-government" characterized the spirit and goal of the newly created ICN.[26] These nursing leaders envisioned an international professional community that not only fostered greater communication among nurses but also deepened their "sympathy" for each other and made them "greater human beings."[27] Although the goals of the ICW and the ICN were similar, the ICN allowed nurses to concentrate on worldwide nursing issues and yet address the general issues all women faced.[28]

The Federation's Eleven-Year History

Dock wrote that the Federation was formed, "quite informally, without a written constitution and almost without rules."[29] Both organizations united in paying dues to the NCW and both appointed two members who chose a fifth person to act as chair and president of the Federation. They selected Adelaide Nutting (1858–1948), Dock's friend and well-known nursing educator, to a five-year term as president. In that position, Nutting represented the membership of the United State's two professional nursing organizations at the NCW and ICW.[30]

The Federation placed the nursing profession in contact with other national and international women's groups interested in social, political, and professional reform. This access allowed nursing leaders in the United States opportunities to explain the tremendous advances achieved in the profession since 1873. In doing so, these leaders hoped to gain allies among other council members for needed nursing legislation. In preparation for the 1902 triennial meeting of the National Council of Women, the Federation was asked to "appoint a representative nurse [to serve] upon a committee whose duty it shall be to bring the National Council of America into closer relations with international movements."[31] The nurse assigned to that committee was to watch for any changes in the public's views on nursing and to note any "practical manifestation of such change," like legislation affecting nursing or speeches and written material referring to nursing.[32] Dock reported that the Federation selected Sophia Palmer, editor of the *AJN,* to represent nursing to that committee. The NCW also requested that an additional nurse be chosen to assist in a worldwide demonstration scheduled for May that year, favoring arbitration and "universal peace." In recognition of nursing's membership within the council, all nurses affiliated with the Federation were eligible to wear the National Council of Women's pin.[33]

Dock wrote in her Federation report that nurses were starting to take an active role in the national council and were meeting women who stood for progress. Dock hoped that all the members of the Federation would become interested in this affiliation so that they would learn what other women were doing and would "educate themselves to hold intelligent opinions on the constantly arising questions" brought before them.[34]

In February 1904, Helena Barnard from St. Joseph, Missouri, a graduate of the Johns Hopkins Hospital School for Nurses, represented the Federation at a meeting of the Executive Council of Women at Indianapolis. Barnard explained to the council the history of the Superintendents' Society and the Associated Alumnae. She stressed the importance of the new legislation already passed in thirteen states that required nurses to complete a systematic course in nurse training and to pass a state examination before they could use the new title of "Registered Nurse." Barnard asked the women's council to support the Federation's continued efforts in creating this legislation to safeguard the public from unscrupulous schools and untrained nurses. She urged them "in conformity with the ever-growing spirit of philanthropy" to join American nurses in their work to "meet the needs of the day."[35] Barnard asked the societies affiliated with the NCW to "support everywhere the nurse in her effort to secure legislation."[36]

In spite of the inroads established by the Federation's membership within the NCW, nursing leaders believed that they could more effectively accomplish their professional goals through the ICN. As early as 1901, members of nursing organizations questioned the efficacy of membership within the NCW. While attending a NCW meeting in 1901, Emma Keating, the Superintendents' Society president and delegate to the NCW, observed that although the work of the NCW was "interesting and instructive," it was too time-consuming for women in nursing who had so much to accomplish in their own profession. Nonetheless, nursing representation continued in the NCW until 1905, when the Federation voted to drop its membership and to join the ICN.[37]

In 1905, the *Washington Post* announced that the American Federation of Nurses had withdrawn from the NCW but had adopted a resolution "providing that the federation affiliate with the International Council of Nurses."[38] Dock supported the drop in the membership because the National Council of Women was ineffective as a national organization: dues were six times higher than those for other national councils, membership responsibilities were an added burden for the already busy officers of the professional nursing organizations, and membership in the ICN brought greater benefits to American nurses. Dock concluded that although membership in the NCW was theoretically desirable, the limited resources of nursing leaders required that the nursing organizations focus their energies on their members' professional concerns. While Dock believed that joining the ICN could be "definitely helpful and useful in an international union of our colleagues," she personally felt that membership within the NCW had enabled them to "come into relation with nurses of other countries," and gave them "status in the great Congresses of Women."[39]

One factor that may also have influenced the Federation's decision to drop the NCW and join the ICN was that eligibility requirements for membership in the ICN had changed. Because individual membership in the ICN gave way to organizational membership, the Federation served as the appropriate vehicle for American nursing to enter the ICN. Dock and others thought it would be too expensive to carry two such international affiliations and, hence, they dropped their NCW membership. Nevertheless, the Federation's membership in the ICN continued the ties American nursing had already established with the early twentieth-century woman's movement.[40]

Organized Nursing's Involvement in the Woman's Movement

Through the Federation, American nurses engaged in the suffrage activities of the late-nineteenth- and early-twentieth-century woman's movement. Support of this issue evolved as nurses learned of the relevance suffrage had to their profession, the health of their patients, and their personal lives. The Federation represented nurses' views on the suffrage question at the international council until the Associated Alumnae in 1911 reorganized as the American Nurses' Association (ANA) and fulfilled that job. At that time, provisions were made for a member from the Superintendents' Society and the newly organized National Organization of Public Health Nursing (NOPHN) to serve on the ANA board. In 1912, the ANA represented America's three nursing organizations at the ICN and endorsed the international professional nursing woman suffrage resolution.[41]

In 1909, at the Federation's second convention, outgoing president Adelaide Nutting addressed the group and spoke of the many advancements achieved within the modern nursing movement.[42] She described the development of postgraduate work in nursing; the growth of nursing practice in areas of district nursing, visiting nursing, and school nursing; the programs to prevent tuberculosis; the establishment of milk stations and dispensaries to prevent infant mortality; and the development of social services in hospitals and dispensaries.[43] Nutting argued that nursing must support the other social movements such as suffrage, prohibition, moral prophylaxis, and peace, explaining that these movements had influenced nursing's development and thus warranted its support.[44] Suffrage, according to Nutting, especially deserved a commitment from the nursing community. She warned the audience that no matter what their individual opinions and preferences might be regarding these movements, they could not afford to remain "ignorant of these matters and of the issues involved in them."[45]

At the Federation's 1909 convention, nurses had an opportunity to demonstrate their commitment to woman suffrage when Lavinia Dock read the resolution referred to as "The Enfranchisement of Women." In spite of many of the speakers' interest in the issue and after a prolonged discussion among the members, however, the Federation failed to endorse woman suffrage; by a vote of forty-eight against and twenty-eight in favor, the four American delegates were instructed to vote against an international woman suffrage resolution at the upcoming International Council of Nurses meeting.[46]

Two years later, Dock wanted to avert another negative vote at the next Congress of Nurses in Cologne, Germany, in August 1912. She highlighted the resolutions to be voted on at that congress in the October 1911 issue of the *AJN*. The projected resolutions dealt with the care of old and infirmed nurses, the endorsement of state registration, the improvement of educational standards, and the recognition of women's vote in shaping "a more just social order."[47] Because the newly reorganized ANA subsumed the representative responsibilities of the Federation at the ICN meetings, Dock hoped that delegates to the ANA convention that year would be given "explicit instructions" by their alumnae associations concerning woman suffrage. Dock wanted to avoid the embarrassment experienced by the "misguided" American delegates at the 1909 ICN conference held in London. This time she wanted the international nursing delegates to be given a clear message that the nurses in the United States supported the international woman suffrage resolution.

Dock's efforts to gain support among nurses for woman suffrage rose as public interest in suffrage increased throughout the United States. As more states granted women full suffrage rights, it seemed to some that woman suffrage was "destined to prevail."[48] In keeping with the increasing demand for suffrage among women and the increasing social awareness among nurses, woman suffrage gained nursing's official approval.

Conclusion

American nurses formed the Federation in 1901 to partake in the progressive activities of the NCW and subsequently the ICW. By the time the Federation held its first meeting in May 1905 in Washington, D.C., at the Superintendents' Society Eleventh Annual Convention, the Federation had already sent delegates to three annual meetings of the NCW, in Buffalo, 1901; Washington, 1902; and Indianapolis, 1904. The Federation had also represented American nursing at the ICW quinquennial held in Berlin in 1904.[49] The Federation represented American nursing's two professional organizations in the NCW until 1905. At that time, nursing leaders felt that it would be more advantageous for the Federation to belong to the ICN than the NCW. The Federation switched its membership from the NCW directly to the ICN. Just as the NCW served as the gatekeeper to the ICW, the Federation became the gatekeeper to the ICN. The Federation continued to represent nursing's two national associations until the ANA in 1912 officially assumed that role, thus ending the life of the American Federation of Nurses. However, during the Federation's brief eleven-year span, American nurses became involved in the ongoing woman's movement and the international social, political, and economic drive to allow women personal and professional choice. The Federation provided a forum in which nursing leaders such as Lavinia Dock, Isabel Hampton Robb, and Adelaide Nutting could successfully argue the case for American nursings' pragmatic involvement with the woman's movement at the beginning of the twentieth century. This eleven-year period reflected the strong influence and determination of the nursing profession to expand its horizons and partake in the reform movement.

Sandra B. Lewenson, EdD, RN
Assistant Professor
College of Nursing
State University of New York
Health Science Center at Brooklyn

133 Mt. Hope Boulevard
Hastings-on-Hudson, N.Y. 10706
Phone: (914) 478-4496

Acknowledgments

This work is adapted from Sandra Lewenson, Taking Charge: Nursing, Suffrage, and Feminism in America, 1873–1920 *(New York: Garland, in press). The author wishes to thank Joan E. Lynaugh for her generous comments and Zeta Omega Westchester-Rockland At Large Chapter of Sigma Theta Tau for their partial support.*

Notes

1. Lavinia Dock, "International Relationships," [Report of] The American Federation of Nurses published in *Eleventh Annual Report of the ASSTSN including Report of the First Meeting of the American Federation of Nurses 1905* (Baltimore, Md.: J. H. Furst Company, 1905), 170.

2. See Nancy F. Cott, *The Grounding of Modern Feminism* (New Haven, Conn.: Yale University Press, 1987), 13; and Nancy F. Cott, "What's in a Name? The Limits of 'Social Feminism'; or, Expanding the Vocabulary of Women's History," *The Journal of American History* 76 (December 1989): 809–29, for the different meanings and ongoing discussion regarding use of feminist terminology. Cott describes the discussions and disagreements among late twentieth-century historians regarding the definition of feminism, feminists, and social feminism. Although I am hesitant to use the term "feminist" to describe Dock's visionary role in the beginning of the twentieth century, I think that individuals (like Dock) and events (like membership in international congresses) were feminist in their actions and activities, even though these terms were not applied or widely used in America until 1913. In addition, I use the term feminist because there are few terms that so conveniently describe, to later twentieth-century readers, those activities of women in the

late nineteenth and early twentieth century who politically challenged male domination and control of women's personal and professional lives. See Sandra Lewenson, "The Relationship Among the Four Professional Nursing Organizations and Woman Suffrage: 1893–1920" (EdD diss., Teachers College, Columbia University, N.Y., 1989, University Microfilms International, order number 9002561), v–vii, and Sandra Lewenson, "The Woman's Nursing and Suffrage Movement, 1893–1920," in *Florence Nightingale and Her Era: A Collection of New Scholarship,* ed. Vern Bullough, Bonnie Bullough, and Marietta Stanton (New York: Garland Publishing, 1990), 123, for discussion regarding the argument that organized nursing be remembered for actively participating in the early twentieth century woman's movement, specifically in its campaign for woman suffrage.

3. Sophia Palmer, Training School Alumnae Associations, *First and Second Annual Conventions of the ASSTSN* (Harrisburg, Pa.: Harrisburg Publishing Co., 1897), 55, The Adelaide Nutting Historical Nursing Collection, The Milbank Memorial Library, Teachers College, Columbia University, N.Y. (hereafter called ANHNC, MML, TC, CU); Susan Reverby, ed., *Annual Conventions ASSTSN* (New York: Garland Publishing Co., 1985), 55.

4. Lena Dufton, ed., *History of Nursing at New York Post-Graduate Medical School and Hospital* (New York: The Alumnae Association, 1944), 71–72; unpublished minutes of the Fourth Annual Convention of the Nurses Associated Alumnae, 16 and 17 September 1901, Mugar Memorial Library, Nursing Archives, American Nurses' Association, Board of Directors Minutes: 1897–1949 (Records of Associated Alumnae of U.S. and Canada, 1897–1912), N87, Boston University, Boston, box 33, p. 70 (hereafter cited as MML–NA); Mary Thornton, along with Miss Healy, was selected by Isabel Hampton Robb to represent the Nurses' Associated Alumnae at the American Federation of Nurses.

5. Dock, "International Relationships," 170.

6. Letter addressed to Miss F. Isaac from the President of the NCW (unsigned), dated 17 December 1898, National League for Nursing, History of Medicine Division, National Library of Medicine, Bethesda, Md. (hereafter cited as NLN, MS. C 274, HMD, NLM), box 6, p. 47. The president of the Superintendents' Society was Isabel McIsaac, however, the letter was addressed to Miss F. Isaac.

7. Ibid.

8. *Seventh Annual Convention of The American Society of Superintendents of Training Schools for Nurses* (Harrisburg, Pa.: Harrisburg Publishing Co., 1900), 29–33, for a discussion in the minutes concerning membership in the NCW; Letter to Miss L. L. Dock from May Wright Sewall, dated 23 February 1900 [summary], in the *Seventh Annual Convention,* 30–32; Extracts from Draft Constitution of International Council of Nurses, *Seventh Annual Convention of the Superintendents' Society,* 110.

9. Ethel Bedford Fenwick, *Seventh Annual Convention,* 111; Josephine Dolan, *Nursing in Society: A Historical Perspective,* 13th ed. (Philadelphia, Pa.: W. B. Saunders Co., 1973), 251, notes that the purpose of the Federation was to afford "membership in the National Council of Women and participation in the proceedings of the I. C. N."

10. Letter dated 4 October 1900, addressed "Dear Madam" from Lavinia Dock, NLN, MS. C 274, HMD, NLM, Bethesda, Md., box 6, p. 44; Second Annual Convention of the Associated Alumnae, 2 May 1899, afternoon session, "Board of Directors Minutes 1897–1929," MML, NA, N 87, Convention proceedings, box 33, folder 1. The unpublished minutes shows none of the discussions or decisions on the subject.

11. Isabel Hampton Robb, "Original Communications: Address of the President," *American Journal of Nursing* 1, no. 2 (November 1900): 103 (hereafter cited as *AJN*).

12. Excerpt of Letter from May Wright Sewall, "Report of the Third Annual Convention of the Associated Alumnae of Trained Nurses," *AJN* 1, no. 1 (October 1900): 76.

13. Comment by Lavinia Dock in the "Report of the Third annual Convention of the Associated Alumnae of Trained Nurses," *AJN* 1, no. 1 (1900): 76.

14. Ibid.; see also unnamed and undated newspaper clipping, "The Nursing World," NLN, MS. C 274, HMD, NLM, Bethesda, Md., box 6, p. 40.

15. Dock, "International Relationships," 170; Elizabeth M. Jamieson and May Sewall, *Trends in Nursing History: Their Relationships to World Events,* 4th ed. (Philadelphia, Pa.: W. B. Saunders Co., 1954), 550; Dock, "The International Council of Nurses," 116.

16. Third Annual Convention of the NAA 3–5 May 1900, "Board of Directors Minutes 1897–1929," MML, NA, N 87, Convention proceedings, box 33, folder 1, pp. 41–59; Letter dated 4 October 1900, addressed "Dear Madam" from Lavinia Dock, NLN, MS. C 274, HMD, NLM, Bethesda, Md., box 6, p. 44, for announcement that affiliation between the Superintendents' Society and the Associated Alumnae for the purpose of entering the National Council of Women was approved; "Report of the Third Annual Convention of the Associated Alumnae of Trained Nurses," *AJN* 1, no. 1 (October 1900): 77. The committee selected to study the affiliation between the Superintendents' Society and the Associated Alumnae included Lavinia Dock from Bellevue; Miss Graham from New York Post-Graduate; Miss Brobson from the University of Pennsylvania; Miss Thornton from the Farrand Training School; and Jessie Breeze from Illinois, who was selected as chair.

17. May Wright Sewall as quoted in the International Council of Women, *Women in a Changing World, The Dynamic Story of the International Council of Women Since 1888* (London: Routledge and Kegan Paul, 1966), 12.

18. Ibid., 3–39, for the history of the International Council of Women between 1888 and 1914.

19. *Women in a Changing World,* 206, for quoted material.

20. Cott, "What's in a Name," 809–29; Robert L. Daniels, *American Women in the 20th Century: The Festival of Life* (San Diego, Calif.: Harcourt Brace Jovanovich, 1987), 33–35; Angela Howard Zophy, "Social Feminism," and "Social Housekeeping," in *Handbook of American Women's History,* ed. Angela Howard Zophy and Frances M. Kavenik (Garland Reference Library of the Humanities V. 696, 1990), 557, 558; Mary I. Wood, *The History of the General Federation of Women's Clubs* (New York: General Federation of Women's Clubs, 1912), 22–40; Frances E. Willard,

Glimpses of Fifty Years: The Autobiography of an American Woman (Chicago, Ill.: Woman's Temperance Publication Association, 1889), 590–92.

21. Fannie Humphries Gafney and Kate Waller Barrett, *Seventh Annual Convention of the American Society of Superintendents of Training Schools for Nurses,* 109.

22. Inez Haynes Irwin, *Angels and Amazons: A Hundred Years of American Women* (Garden City, N.Y.: Doubleday, Doran and Company, 1933), Appendix 445; Irwin wrote that over 150,000 women had attended the sixty sessions, which included 600 speakers, at the Chicago World's Exposition in 1893. *International Council of Women Handbook,* 2nd ed. (1899). *Handbook of the International Congress—Program of Quinquennial Meetings of the International Council of Women,* 2nd ed. (1899), 57, located in envelope marked p. 13, NLN, MS. C 274, HMD, NLM, box 6; Cott, *Grounding of Modern Feminism,* 255; and D. C. Bridges, *A History of the International Council of Nurses, 1899–1964* (Philadelphia, Pa.: Lippincott, 1967), for general description of the International Council of Nurses and of the relationship between American nursing organizations and the woman movement through their affiliation with the ICN.

23. Any connection between the International Congress of Women and the Nurses Congress at the 1893 Columbian Exposition is speculative at this time; further investigation is needed to clarify the relationship between the two events. Nevertheless, the connection between the two events was alluded to by the editor of the *American Journal of Nursing,* who wrote in September 1901 that "our national and international fellowships and affiliations with other bodies of women are a direct offspring" of the Congress held at the Columbian Exposition. See, "The Editor," *AJN* 1, no. 12 (September 1901): 941. The September issue was devoted to the planned events and biographies of those in attendance at the Pan American Exposition held in September 1901.

24. Dock, "International Relationships," 169.

25. Ibid.

26. Margaret Breay and Ethel Gordon Fenwick, *History of the International Council of Nurses 1899–1925* (Geneva: The I. C. N., 1931), 59.

27. Ibid., 59; Lavinia L. Dock and Isabel Maitland Stewart, *A Short History of Nursing From the Earliest Times to the Present Day* (New York: G. P. Putnam's Sons, 1931), 344–46, for description of the ICN; *Fourth Annual Convention of the American Society of Superintendents of Training Schools for Nurses* (Harrisburg, Pa.: Harrisburg Publishing Co., 1897), 13, 37; Reverby, *Annual Conventions,* 13, 37, for letter sent to the Superintendents' Society and the selection of delegates Draper and Smith; and *Fifth Annual Convention of the American Society of Superintendents of Training Schools for Nurses* (Harrisburg, Pa.: Harrisburg Publishing Co., 1898), 11; Reverby, *Annual Conventions,* 11, for Snively's concern for cost of sending delegates.

28. Lavinia Dock, "The International Council of Nurses," *AJN* 1, no. 2 (November 1900): 114. The Matron's Council had formed a Provisional Committee to form the International Council of Nurses: Dock includes the constitution written by the provisional committee and adopted in July 1900 in London. Editorial, "1899–July 1929," *The ICN* 9, no. 3 (July 1929): 14–15. According to Dock's editorial, the ICN was considered the oldest among the international councils to be established by a professional group of workers. Other international professional councils to

form included the International Dental Federation in 1900, the International Society of Surgeons in 1902, the International Pharmaceutical Federation in 1912, the International Association of Midwives in 1925, and the International Professional Medical Association in 1926.

29. Dock, "International Relationships," 170.

30. Unpublished minutes of Superintendents' Society, dated Detroit June 1902 and signed L. L. Dock, secretary, NLN, MS. C 274, HMD, NLM, box 2, Exhibit 3a, p. 99; Lystra Gretter, *Ninth Annual Convention of the ASSTSN* (Harrisburg, Pa.: Harrisburg Publishing Co., 1902), 6–7; Lavinia Dock, Report from committee on affiliation with the National Council of Women at the Eighth Annual Meeting of the ASSTSN, held on 16 September 1901, NLN, MS. C 274, HMD, NLM, box 2, Exhibit 3a, p. 96.

31. Lavinia L. Dock, "Official Reports of Societies: The American Federation of Nurses," *AJN* 2, no. 5 (February 1902): 377.

32. Ibid.

33. Ibid.

34. Ibid.

35. Report of The American Federation of Nurses, *AJN* 4, no. 8 (May 1904): 619.

36. Ibid., 621.

37. Emma J. Keating, Report as Delegate to the National Council of Women, *Proceedings of the Eighth Annual Convention of the ASSTSN* (held in 1901) (Harrisburg, Pa.: Harrisburg Publishing Co., 1902), 17–18. The American delegates who attended the International Congress of Nurses in Buffalo in 1901 represented the many different training-school alumnae associations and nursing associations. That year Isabel McIsaac was the president of the Congress of Nurses.

38. "Busy Day for Nurses," *Washington Post,* May 1905 (date unknown), NLN, MS.C 274, HMD, NLM, box 6, p. 84; Lucy Ridgely Seymer, *A General History of Nursing* (New York: Macmillan Co., 1933), 270. American nursing had attended the ICN's first Quinquennial meeting in Berlin, Germany, in 1904, and was one of three countries (the other two were Great Britain and Germany) to have a national organization affiliated. However, Seymer does not mention the American Federation of Nurses.

39. Dock, "International Relationships," 176.

40. Dock, "International Relationships," 169–176; Unpublished Minutes of Council Meeting of the Superintendents' Society, 30 April 1905, NLN, MS. C 274, HMD, NLM, box 2, Exhibit 3b, 187–88. In preparation for the Superintendents' Society Convention, a joint meeting with the Associated Alumnae constituting the first meeting of the American Federation of Nurses was planned for the 1905 annual convention. There they planned to discuss affiliation with the International Council of Nurses and possible plans to withdraw from the National Council of Women.

41. Editorial Comment, "The Chicago Conventions," *AJN* 12, no. 10 (July 1912): 770; and Unpublished Minutes of Council Meeting of the Superintendents' Society, 12 January 1912, held in Nutting's office, NLN, MS. C 274, HMD, NLM, box 2, Exhibit 3b, 254; Mary Roberts, *American Nursing: History and Interpretation* (New York: Macmillan Co.), 79; Lewenson, *Relationship Among the Four Professional*

Nursing Organizations, 159–60. Neither the Federation nor the ANA included the National Association of Colored Graduate Nurses (NACGN), founded in 1908, in their activities. However, the NACGN sent their own representatives to the ICN.

42. The Superintendents' Society, the Associated Alumnae, and the American Federation of Nurses held joint sessions during the first week of June 1909 in St. Paul, Minnesota. It was the Superintendents' Society's Fifteenth Annual Meeting, the Associated Alumnae's Twelfth Annual Meeting, and the American Federation of Nurses' second meeting (their first meeting was held in 1905).

43. Adelaide Nutting, President's opening remarks at the Second Meeting of the AFN, *Fifteenth Annual Report of ASSTSN including Report of the Second Meeting of the AFN: 1909* (Baltimore, Md.: J. H. Furst, 1910), 101–8.

44. Moral prophylaxis related to the self-regulation of one's moral code, which would inhibit sexual activity outside of marriage for men and women. Many believed that this would stop the spread of venereal diseases and reduce prostitution. Historian Janet James defined social hygiene as a "euphemism for VD prevention" and morality as "abolition of prostitution." See Lavinia L. Dock, *Hygiene and Morality: A Manual for Nurses and Others, Giving an Outline of the Medical, Social, and Legal Aspects of Venereal Disease,* in *A Lavinia Dock Reader,* ed. Janet James (New York: Garland Publishing, 1985), 90–91.

45. Nutting, 106.

46. *Fifteenth Annual Report of ASSTSN,* 215; The American Federation of Nurses voted for Annie Goodrich (1866–1954), Isabel Hampton Robb, Jane Delano (1858–1919), and Nancy (?) Cadmus to represent the Federation at the 1909 International Council of Nurses in London.

47. Lavinia L. Dock, "Nursing News and Announcements: International," *AJN* 12, no. 1 (October 1911): 58.

48. "Book Reviews: Women in Public Affairs," *AJN* 13, no. 5 (February 1913): 495. This review was excerpted from "The Progress of the World," in the *American Review of Reviews* for January 1913, and it referred to the Progressive party's work in woman suffrage.

49. Unpublished minutes of Superintendents' Society, dated Detroit June 1902 and signed L. L. Dock, secretary, NLN, MS. C 274, HMD, NLM, box 2, Exhibit 3a, p. 99; Gretter, *Ninth Annual Convention of the ASSTSN,* 6–7.

Caring without Politics: Lessons from the First Nurses of the North and South

QUINCEALEA BRUNK
The University of Alabama School of Nursing
The University of Alabama at Birmingham

When the Civil War broke out in 1861, no one anticipated the response to a call for volunteers to serve in the military to come from women. A woman's sphere was clearly designated to be the home during the antebellum years, and society expected this separatist philosophy of gender roles to hold true in wartime as well.[1] However, shortly after the firing on Fort Sumter and President Lincoln's call for volunteers, the women of both the North and the South took it upon themselves to answer a unique call to duty. They sensed the need to care for the sick and wounded long before the military hospital system was well established and took their monopoly of knowledge about caring for the sick to those who needed it most.

The United States Sanitary Commission and local Ladies' Aid Societies began relief work in the North as soon as the war broke out, but individual women took on the responsibility of nursing the sick and wounded soldiers. From the beginning, the South relied entirely on volunteerism and the patriotic spirit of its women to care for Confederate soldiers. As the war continued, the demands for volunteers to tend to the wounded exceeded the supply of women with even a meager amount of training. Thus, amateur caregivers constituted the greatest portion of nurses for both sides of the conflict throughout the war.[2]

Dorothea Dix is traditionally credited with becoming the first volunteer when she offered her services as the Superintendent of Women Nurses to the Union government, but historical evidence suggests otherwise. Moreover, the exclusive focus on Dix's key role in the supervision of nurses for the North has overshadowed the early contributions made by lesser-known women nurses. This account corrects the historical record and broadens the story to bring to life the real women who answered the call for volunteers—in both the North and South.

Nursing History Review 2 (1994): 119–136.

The Union's First Nurse

Adeline Blanchard Tyler was born to Jeremiah and Mary (Gowan) Blanchard on 8 December 1805 in Billerica, Massachusetts. Little is known of her early life; she was educated at Boston academies, and she married John Tyler in 1826. The Tylers had no children, and Mrs. Tyler became active in the Episcopal church, devoting many hours to charitable work. After her husband's death in 1853 she became a deaconess in the Episcopal church, traveling to Europe to take training as a nurse at the Kaiserswerth Institute. Upon her return to Boston, she resumed her charitable activities in the role of deaconess and performed nursing duties for the sick of the parish.[3]

Early in the summer of 1856, Tyler's life underwent a major change when she received a letter requesting her services as principal for a small infirmary attached to St. Andrew's Church in Baltimore. Although her roots were in Boston, Tyler answered the call and had the infirmary ready to accept patients within a matter of days after her arrival in mid-September 1856. The infirmary quickly gained a reputation for excellent and charitable care but was plagued by financial adversity from its first opening. Although it remained independent for about a year, the small infirmary was eventually amalgamated with the Church Home Society in Baltimore.

Although reluctant to take on the responsibility assigned her, Tyler became the head deaconess of the Church Home Infirmary. She had several deaconesses in training under her supervision and managed most of the financial affairs of the institution. The position was not without its difficulties, however. Questions and complaints of excess charity on Tyler's part were raised before Bishop Whittingham on several occasions.[4]

As financial adversity and conflicts continued, the governing board for the Church Home decided that the hospital required new management. Rev. R. Clarence Hall was appointed warden on 25 January 1860. Tyler was given the news that he had been placed in command of the Church Home a week later in a letter:

> You will perceive that this action requires at least *in form* a reorganization of the internal government of the Institution. . . . Waiving at present the powers with which I am clothed as vice-rector I earnestly solicit you and the ladies associated with you to continue to render the services.[5]

Apparently irritated with the new management structure forced on her, Adeline Tyler submitted her resignation as chief deaconess of the Church Home Infirmary on 14 February, requesting leave to retire and continue the work of training the subordinates at the deaconesses' home. On 5 March 1860, her resignation was acknowledged and accepted. Although retired from hospital work, Tyler remained active in preparing others for service as the crisis of the Union mounted.

> For the last year of peace and the early months of war she had lived in the deaconesses' home instructing her apprentice deaconesses, nursing the sick and destitute in their own houses, caring for Baltimore children "orphaned or worse than orphaned," visiting the prisons. For a time, when a typhoid epidemic filled the infirmary with more patients than her fellow-deaconesses could care for, she was back at the Church Home nursing. But it must have seemed to her that her greatest usefulness was past. In fact it was to come.[6]

Wartime Activities

On 19 April 1861, the Federal soldiers in command of Fort Sumter had already surrendered to the Confederate forces, and President Lincoln had called for 75,000 volunteers to support the standing army. The 6th Massachusetts Volunteer Regiment was the first regiment ready to travel to Washington, D.C., to defend the nation's capital. En route they passed through Baltimore, where they were mobbed by angry crowds. At least two men were killed in the attack, and several others were wounded.[7] Because Maryland was a border state, sentiments for the war varied among the people. Although this tension did not deter Tyler from her vision of duty, its consequences were to plague her throughout her time in Baltimore.

Tyler received the news of the attack on the troops from her home state. She learned of the wounded men's imprisonment in the city police station from Alexander Fulton late in the afternoon of 19 April 1861. She immediately began to make preparations to care for the wounded men in her home. She set out for the police station in her carriage as darkness set in on the wrecked streets of Baltimore. When she arrived, she was denied admission, and the officers were openly contemptuous of her notions of caring for the wounded men. After several attempts to gain entry, she informed the chief officer that she would contact the governor of Massachusetts if she was not allowed to treat the "prisoners" humanely and dress their wounds.[8] With this threat, the resistance ceased, and she was allowed to enter the station.

Tyler persuaded the chief officer to permit the two most seriously wounded men to be moved to her own home, going so far as to encourage the police to send a guard to her house if they did not trust her. The two wounded men were smuggled to her home in a furniture van after ten o'clock that night. As one account noted, "A brave heart indeed it required for a lady to be left alone in such a place, at such an hour, and amid such painful surroundings, but she was more than equal to the emergency."[9] Both prisoners stayed under Tyler's roof for about a month until they recuperated sufficiently to travel and rejoin their company.

In the midst of all the excitement in Baltimore, Dorothea Dix was just making her way to Washington, D.C., to offer her services as the Superintendent of Women Nurses. Her train, which passed through Baltimore three hours after the mobbing, was slightly delayed.[10] Thus, Adeline Blanchard Tyler can justly be given the honor of being the "first nurse" to treat Union forces in the Civil War.

The brutal mobbing of soldiers in the streets of Baltimore illustrated the mixed feelings of the people as war came to the nation. This frightening display of public sentiment soon led to the resignation of several of the deaconesses training under Tyler's supervision at the school on Howard Street. The exodus of the trainees forced the school to close, leaving Tyler jobless. Although she was past the age specified for volunteer nurses under Dix, her training and experience were seen as assets to the Union forces; she was officially asked to share her expertise. Because she was still committed to her church responsibilities, Tyler sought approval from the bishop for her assignments throughout the war. In her annual report to the bishop dated St. Matthew's Day (September) 1861, Tyler stated:

> I have been asked by Miss Dix, Superintendent of the nursing department in the Government Hospitals to take a position in a Hospital where I could introduce the services of a band of my co-workers. This I defer to you and our excellent chaplain holding myself ready in my abilities to engage in any work that you may deem needful to accomplish the one great end, the glory of God and the Salvation of Souls.[11]

The bishop apparently approved of the assignment, for Tyler took charge of the Camden Street Hospital in Baltimore later that month. At fifty-five years of age, Adeline Blanchard Tyler undertook the task that would constitute her life's achievement. She faced multiple trials that required a great deal of endurance, but she possessed the experience and fortitude necessary for the leadership charge. Still, in her early days in this demanding position, she had some doubts regarding her abilities. She detailed some of her frustrations at Camden Street in a letter to her sister.

> The sick, the wounded and the dying are all around; jealousies exist among the subordinate nurses; difficulties arise between physicians and nurses; com-

plaints made alike by nurses and patients; ceaseless inquiries and interruptions coming from visitors and sub-officials; all these together with the feeling of grave responsibility make the position one calling for the most patient endurance and the wisest and promptest administration.[12]

In the spring of 1862, Tyler was honored by the Massachusetts Legislature for the care she had given to the wounded men of the 6th Massachusetts Volunteer Regiment. The honors paid her, however, did not prevent some from criticizing her work at the hospital in Baltimore. Tyler retained her position at the Camden Street Hospital only until the summer of 1862. The scant information regarding her termination comes from a communication from a Dr. Atkinson, who had first met Tyler while she was in charge of the Church Home.

When the City was occupied by United States troops a large Hospital was established on Camden Street at the head of which Mrs. Tyler was placed. The impression prevailed that the Confederate wounded were not supplied with proper comforts; and at the request of some of our friends I went to Mrs. Tyler and asked whether if we sent to the Hospital articles of Luxury suited for sick men we might depend upon their being appropriated to our friends. She replied: "Doctor, I do not ask whether he comes from the North or South. I do for him the best I can, and supply his wants from any stores that I have in my possession. If your friends are willing to send supplies for the wounded with that understanding I shall be glad to have them. If I am required to make distinctions I must do without the supplies." I answered. "Mrs. Tyler, we are perfectly willing to trust you, and the supplies shall be sent." This was done and Mrs. Tyler administered the Hospital on the principle of perfect impartiality. I am sorry to add that as a consequence she was turned out of her place, after a few months, as a Rebel sympathizer! as you know she was a devoted Unionist. But she met the fate usual to those who in times of excitement act on principle.[13]

Upon her discharge from Camden Street Hospital, Tyler returned to Boston for a rest. She was unable to stay idle for very long, however, and soon she began recruiting women to serve as nurses. In late August 1862, Tyler wrote to Bishop Whittingham in Baltimore requesting to be placed back on duty. Her timing of the letter was opportune, for the bishop had just received a request for nurses from the chaplain at the Chester U.S. Hospital in Pennsylvania. After asking Tyler's permission to forward her name, the bishop responded to the chaplain on 30 August 1862.

My Chief Deaconess, Mrs. Adeline Tyler . . . yesterday notified me that she was ready for duty again. But she is rather a Superintendent of Nurses, than a mere

> nurse. She is very likely, however, to be able to bring others with her, deaconesses or Probationers.[14]

Just prior to leaving for Pennsylvania in September 1862, Tyler communicated her feelings about the new assignment to the bishop.

> If I had a band of associates trained to the work of a Hospital I would Cheerfully go to Chester but the responsibility of training under the pressure of work in our Hospitals without the aid or even Charitable Considerations of a Surgeon has been in my experience a fearful task. . . . I have several applications from ladies desirous to work with me—my objection is my individuality which makes my position so prominent that if I could avoid it I would like to, nothing but the cry of suffering humanity can induce my voluntary taking such a charge. I am ready to follow your wishes to work in any place you esteem the most useful.[15]

In a letter to her sister a week later, she states, "My present intention is to only remain so long as to systematize their labors and then be returning to New York to meet you and Ellen."[16] However, her time in Pennsylvania was to be longer than she had anticipated. Her arrival at Chester Hospital was greeted with opposition from a group of "ladies," and a great deal of work to be done in the large, one-story barracks hospital that extended a fourth of a mile on each side of an open field. Although required to make rounds only once a day, she usually performed the duty in both the morning and the evening in an attempt to set a stable routine for the facility.

> My post seems to be one of plain duty just now, bringing order out of chaos, and thus far, very unsatisfactorily. I hope to make more progress next week. I have met with all sorts of discouragements. The greatest of these is coming in contact with a band of ladies who were turned from the Hospital before I took charge. I have endeavored to keep out of their contest, and so far have succeeded, although my name is continually brought before the public, as the organ of action employed on "Their premises" as they contend. The Surgeon General will be here tomorrow, and settle the difficulty I trust. If he can make peace between the officers in charge and the ladies I shall hope to be released from my position. Yesterday we received 250 sick and wounded men, 24 of whom are Confederates. . . . They bear marks of privations such as our men have not endured. We have now about a thousand men, some very ill but more convalescing.[17]

Whether the problem with the band of "ladies" was solved in October is unknown, but Tyler was still on duty at Chester Hospital in the spring of

1863. Her communications with her sister over the spring and summer intimate that they were expecting Chester Hospital to be closed by fall, after the present inmates were restored to health. Although the hospital closed that summer, she was not released from duty; instead, she took up a similar post at the Naval School Hospital in Annapolis, Maryland, on 6 July 1863.[18]

Extra care was needed at the Naval School Hospital because many of the patients were Union soldiers who had just been returned from southern prisons. Tyler's responsibilities were varied, including overseeing the diet, dressings, and medicines for the sick and wounded. She began a diary of personal observations and work-related impressions while assigned to Annapolis, but the demands of duty evidently caused her to abandon the cumbersome task of regular entries after just a few weeks.

The sparse entries reveal continued challenges for Tyler; she arrived in Annapolis and reported for duty on Monday (6 July 1863). The entry dated two days later poignantly described the situation at the hospital.

> Went to the Hospital again—learned that several of the nurses had resigned—called a meeting of the remaining four—all of whom are satisfied to remain. We have quarters assigned us in an isolated position—four houses, each containing six rooms, are appropriated to our use. Some repairs are to be made and some painting done, before we can occupy them. Dr. V[anderkeif] has sent to Washington for a Lady who, I hope, will act as an assistant to me, for my duties look so extensive that I almost shrink from attempting what my humble capacity is able to accomplish. I trust in humble confidence to be directed in my thoughts, words and deeds for the comforting of these entrusted to my care and for the furtherance of God's glory.[19]

Tyler's prayers for an assistant were answered, but not before some of her remaining nurses became ill, and on Monday, 13 July, she discovered that one of the four remaining nurses had resigned without telling her. This disappointment was offset by two developments: a hospital official's request that his wife be employed as a nurse, and the promise of an assistant. The following day, her assistant, Miss Hall, arrived and Tyler attempted to "interest her in the different Departments." The younger woman began her duties in Section I the following morning.[20] Later that week, Tyler received letters from three of her former co-workers stating their willingness to come to Annapolis to continue the work for which they had been trained. Although it is not clear that she took their offer of help, Tyler's description of continuing concerns would lead one to suspect that she gratefully accepted.

> Friday [17 July 1863]—we are all worrying through this day trying to make provision for some 375 more patients just from the field. Our demand far exceeds our supply of provisions. All the nurses except one are sick and that one must attend to her fellow-workers. So Miss Hall and myself are the only ones to look after the patients.[21]

Early one morning in August, as she was leaving to perform her rounds, Tyler fell and fractured her shoulder. She was taken to a nearby home where she was cared for until she was able to return to duty in mid-September. She returned to her post at the Naval School Hospital but suffered from continued fatigue under the burden of responsibility. In a letter to her sister in December, Tyler expressed her wish to join her on the European trip, but the anticipated arrival of several hundred paroled prisoners detained her in Annapolis. She wrote, "Much as I desire their release my heart beats with horror for the awful sight of suffering they will present."[22]

The remainder of the winter of 1863–1864 was a particularly trying one for Tyler, for in her correspondence with her sister she expressed her desire to be back among her friends so that she could rest and restore her energies. Her lack of enthusiasm is apparent in a letter written 27 February 1864.

> We are just now relieved from the duty of nursing by the refusal of exchange of prisoners by Jefferson Davis, should he continue in his determination we shall be relieved from this post and I shall never take another task so responsible in any emergency not because I feel unwilling, but because I am incompetent for the work.[23]

Tyler continued her labors throughout the winter and into the spring before seeking release from her post because of failing health. Although she felt "incompetent for the work" toward the end of her service, Tyler's contribution to the aims of Union nurses cannot be overstated. Not only had she been the first to serve the Union; she also demonstrated remarkable fortitude in the face of dissension and exhaustion. She used her experience to organize other nurses in managing the care rendered to thousands of sick and wounded soldiers. Tyler resigned her position at the Naval School Hospital on 27 May 1864, and prepared to join her sister in Europe.

After traveling through Europe for about eighteen months, Tyler returned to the United States in November 1865, at least somewhat rested by her trip abroad. Her charitable works continued, and in 1868 she became associated with the Midnight Mission in New York City. A year later she was named "Lady Superintendent" for the mission, caring for the destitute and sick of that city until she resigned and retired in 1872. She died of breast cancer on 9 January 1875, at her home in Needham, Massachusetts, at the age of sixty-nine, and was buried in Mount Auburn Cemetery in Cambridge.[24]

The First Nurse for the Confederacy

Like the women of the North, the women of the South responded to the call for volunteers, but their goal was to defend the Confederacy. Although some women were able to secretly enlist in the army, most women remained at home to oversee farms and plantations and to supply the troops with necessities. Some left their homes and cared for the sick and wounded in hospitals. Although the first such instance of volunteer caregiving is not carefully documented in southern war annals, it is known that women in Memphis began service in the first month of armed hostilities.

Sallie Chapman Gordon Law was born in Wilkes County, North Carolina, on 27 August 1805, to Chapman and Charity (King) Gordon. She attributed her "martial blood" to her ancestors, especially her father, who had served in the Revolutionary War under Generals Marion and Sumter. Her brother, Wyley J. Gordon, was an officer during the war of 1812, and many of her close relatives served in the Confederate army.[25]

Little is known about Law's early childhood. On her marriage to Dr. John S. Law on 28 June 1825, she moved to Forsythe, Georgia, and in 1834 the Laws moved to Columbia, Tennessee. After the death of her husband in 1844, Law took her seven children to Memphis, hoping to secure better advantages for them. Memphis was her home for the remainder of her life. She was characterized as a self-reliant, charitable, and devout Presbyterian.

Wartime Activities

Sallie Chapman Gordon Law became known as the "mother of the Confederacy" by thoroughly identifying with the southern cause. Although she had more than two score of kinsmen in active service, she "chafed at having only one son to lend to the Confederate armies and was quick to dedicate her own energies to the aid of her section."[26]

When the war broke out she was swift to organize relief work with other women "to care for the sick Confederate soldiers passing through Memphis." Law was acclaimed the first and only president of the Southern Mothers' Society and Hospital at the organization's meeting in a local parlor. The twelve-bed hospital was operational on Second Street by mid-April 1861, when the ladies of the Memphis organization were asked to care for wounded soldiers in General Thomas Carmichael Hindman's command.[27] The mid-April date of the hospital's opening and Law's documentation of nursing activities only days after the war began support the contention that Law was the first Confederate nurse.

Before the summer had passed the hospital outgrew its quarters. The Southern Mothers' Society acquired the Irving Block building, which increased the hospital's capacity to more than four hundred beds. In the early days of the hospital, the ladies of Memphis supplied needed materials from their own stores, but as the undertaking grew Law appealed to other donors for the money and supplies needed to care for the sick and wounded soldiers. Her appeals proved so effective that soon a surplus of supplies was available.

> In our hospital we had many articles not then needed, domestic wines, lemons, pickles, and clothing, and I proposed taking them to our sick soldiers at Columbus, Kentucky. I had large boxes packed and carried them to the hospital there. I made the second trip a few weeks later with more supplies for the sick.[28]

During her second trip to Columbus, Law and her lady companions were eyewitnesses to the Battle of Belmont.[29] Law recounted a great deal of excitement over this particular battle. Not only was her son marched out under General Cheatham's command as she watched from the pavement, but the steamer that was housing the ladies during their visit was used to transport the injured, including the wounded General William H. Jackson, to safety.

Watching the battle from the pilothouse on the shore, one of the other ladies observed, "[the Confederates are] getting whipped; see, our men are running." With a fierce sense of patriotism and enthusiasm for the justness of the southern cause, Law replied, "We are not whipped; our men are going to the river for water." But the soldiers had in fact run out of ammunition and had retreated to the riverbank for protection until supplies could be transported from the Columbus side of the river. Word of Law's comment soon spread to the soldiers, becoming an oft-repeated slogan: "Not running, but going for water."[30]

The battle was recorded as a great victory for the Confederate army, as hundreds of the Union soldiers were left on the battlefield. Further excitement was recorded as high-ranking officers and physicians came to see

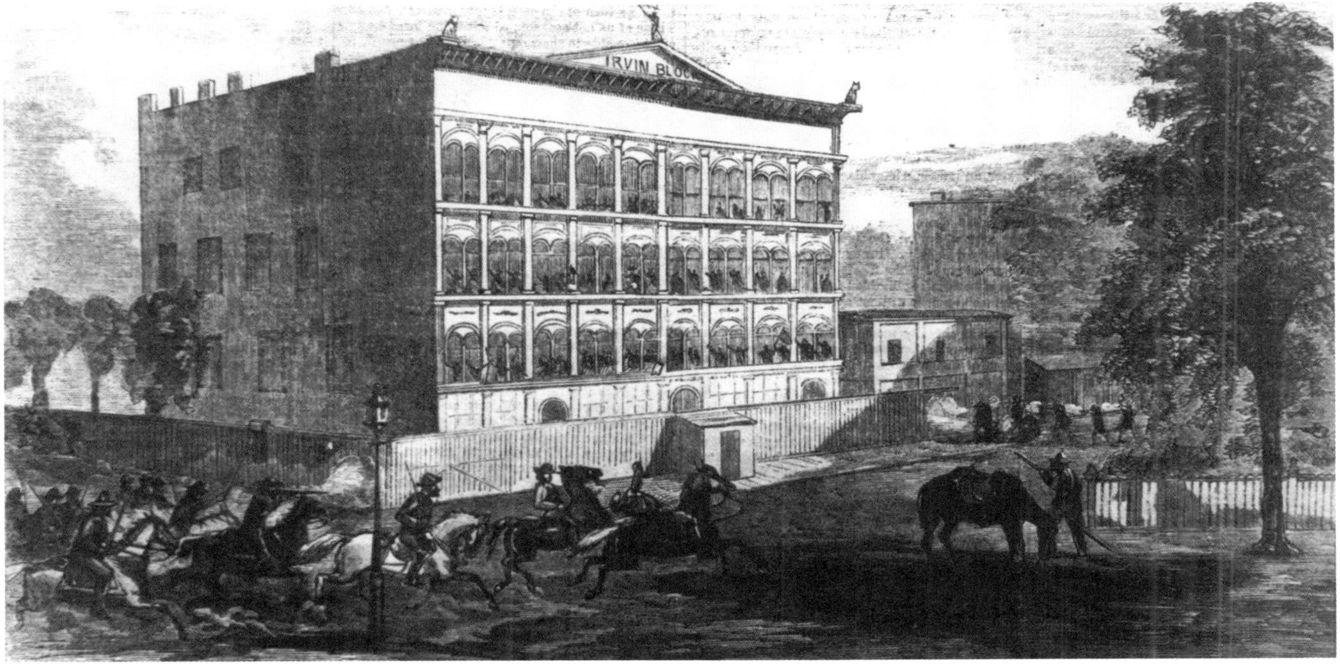

The Irving Block, a commercial building facing Court Square, was used as a Confederate Hospital in Memphis until June 1862, when Union forces occupying the city converted it into a prison. From *Harper's Weekly* (10 Sept. 1864) 8:588. (Courtesy of the Memphis and Shelby County Room, Memphis Shelby County Public Library and Information Center)

General Jackson later in the day. Law went to the hospital to see if anything could be done for the wounded. Despite her strong southern ties and sympathies, her heart was touched by a Union officer who was mortally wounded: "At sight of the wounded man I lost sight of the enemy of my country. I made a glass of lemonade and fed him with a spoon, as one arm was cut off and the other paralyzed."[31] Sitting with the officer, she inquired as to whether he had a wife. When he answered affirmatively, she requested that General Polk send for the wife, who by two o'clock the next afternoon was at the officer's bedside.

Shortly after the battle at Belmont, Law returned to Memphis, where she found much work to be done at her own hospital.

> Boat loads of the Belmont wounded were sent to the hospitals at Memphis. Our Southern Mothers' Hospital in the Irving block was then moved to the Overton Hospital, where we all nursed and worked together, not only our own dear, wounded soldiers, but many Federal prisoners, nursed with the same care, and receiving the same treatment as our own soldiers.[32]

Although Law gives no details of the intervening period, the care of the sick and wounded soldiers and prisoners continued at the Southern Mothers' Hospital. At one time the hospital housed three hundred measles cases and many of the wounded after the Battle of Shiloh. Despite the fact that the hospital cared for soldiers from the North and the South, the Southern Mothers' Hospital was closed when Union troops occupied Memphis. In the brief time that the Southern Mothers' Hospital was operational, more than two thousand soldiers were cared for, with a mortality rate of less than 4 percent.[33]

Although the hospital closed, Law's usefulness and influence did not go unchanneled. As she prepared to leave Memphis to go further into the safety of the Confederacy, Law learned that her brother, G. W. Gordon, was being held prisoner on a boat anchored in the middle of the Mississippi River. She spent the day along the riverbank trying to get permission to see him. At five o'clock that afternoon she obtained permission from a Union officer to be allowed on board.

> On reaching the boat, it was filled with Confederate officers, prisoners from Johnson's Island, bound for Vicksburg to be exchanged. I found my brother very ill. He told me he had not tasted food for ten days; nothing but the coarse food that a well man could hardly eat, was given him. The surgeon in charge begged me, if possible, to try and send some chickens to make chicken broth for him, and to try to send a prescription for him, for he had not a particle of

medicine of any sort to give the sick under his charge, over a hundred sick men, all officers.[34]

After spending the night on board the boat to be near her brother, Law returned to the city and had the needed medicine and chickens sent to the boat, along with other comforts for her brother. She also promised her brother that she would meet him in Vicksburg to nurse him back to health. She left Memphis the following morning, traveling sixty miles before nightfall, only to learn that her brother had died within ten minutes of arriving in Vicksburg.[35]

Although the Southern Mothers' Hospital had been shut down, money still remained in the hospital's treasury. Compelled to continue their support for the southern cause, the ladies of the hospital society purchased quinine, morphine, and opium to be distributed to other Confederate hospitals. Law carried these drugs to LaGrange, Georgia, on her person. While in Georgia she went about the various hospitals to render whatever aid she could, assisting in the care of the wounded after various battles. She also made daily rounds of the hospital wards to distribute eggnog and coffee.

Exactly when Law left LaGrange and resumed her nursing activities in Columbus, Georgia, is unclear. After returning to Columbus, she heard of the terrible destitution in General Joseph E. Johnston's division in northwest Georgia.

> Hundreds, yes, thousands of soldiers having to sit up all night round a log fire, for want of a blanket. . . . I went directly to a Ladies' Aid Society, where a number of patriotic women of that city [Columbus] were at work for the soldiers. I told what I had heard of the suffering, for want of blankets, by the soldiers, and made an appeal to them for aid, telling them if they would furnish the blankets, I would go in person to Dalton and distribute them to the soldiers.[36]

Law left for Dalton on Christmas night 1863, arriving at three o'clock in the morning. She was warmly received by Dr. John Erskine, an old friend from Memphis. Over the next few days Law distributed the blankets and clothing she had brought with her, and even an overcoat that she had been saving as a relic of the war. Upon returning to Columbus, she wrote for several newspapers, describing what she had seen, and made public appeals for donations for the relief of the soldiers at Dalton.

> I went out and in one hour I collected twenty-five hundred dollars from the business houses, and laid it all out in the Columbus factories for jeans and

> course cloth with which the ladies made comfortable coverings, (the soldiers being in winter quarters.) The women and children worked night and day, and in ten days I returned to the army in Dalton with seven large dry goods boxes, one for Tennessee, one for Kentucky, one for Mississippi, one for Louisiana, one for Arkansas, one for Missouri, and one for Texas, all packed with five hundred and thirty blankets and coverings, and sixteen hundred pairs of socks, for the soldiers.[37]

During a second visit to Dalton, Law and her lady companions were treated like royalty by the military officials. They were invited to dine with the generals and were honored with parties. General Johnston even ordered a grand parade of thirty thousand "bronzed" but tattered soldiers in honor of her mission to his soldiers. This distinction reportedly was afforded to no other woman in the Confederacy, not even Mrs. Jefferson Davis.[38]

In all of her travels during the war, Sallie Chapman Law paid her own expenses, never receiving so much as a railroad pass to carry out her good deeds of relief and nursing.

> [M]y whole heart and thoughts and deepest sympathies were all absorbed in the destiny of my people, in this fratricidal war. My oppressed, my bleeding countrymen, for that just cause I would have died, could that sacrifice have brought peace, instead of a surrender, in which all was lost, save honor.[39]

As the war drew to a close, Law returned to her home in Memphis to spend her remaining years. She occupied her time in the company of her associates from the war days, marking graves and erecting monuments to the brave soldiers of the Confederacy. In May 1889, with the Southern Mothers' Association at its nucleus, the Confederate Historical Association was formed. It was one of the first organizations to recognize the historical legacy of the Confederacy, and the only one to which Jefferson Davis belonged.[40]

In 1892, at the age of eighty-seven, Law complied with the requests of friends and family by writing about her war experiences. Stating that all the incidents of her wartime experiences would have filled a book, Law instead wrote a sixteen-page pamphlet, pleading old age and lack of strength.

> Still memories of suffering, blood, and tears at the bedside of the wounded, dying soldier, is indelibly stamped on the walls of memory, and will probably last until the dreams of this fitful checkered life are over. . . . I have had the honor of being called the "Mother of the Confederacy," a compliment I esteem higher than any that could be conferred upon me.[41]

In the last year of her life, Law was unable to go out in public and failed quickly in the final two months. She died on 28 June 1894, at eighty-nine years of age, with her children at her bedside, at Idlewild, a suburb of Memphis.[42]

Summary

When the lives of the two women who were first to respond as nurses to their country's emergency are compared, more similarities than differences emerge. The clinical and moral imperatives they faced overrode any political considerations. Tyler and Law were both in their mid-fifties and widowed by the time the war broke out in 1861. Both women were educated, probably beyond the normal levels of their era. Although little is known of Law's early life, her organizational aptitude and later writings indicate that she must have had some education in her early years. Further, her actions on behalf of securing better advantages for her children suggest that she valued the educational possibilities and artistic diversity afforded in the city of Memphis.

Both women had some experience in nursing and in managing affairs for large groups or households. Tyler acquired formal training in nursing at the Kaiserswerth Institute, and Law's experience was undoubtedly gained by caring for her seven children. While Tyler was managing an infirmary and training school in Baltimore, Law was managing a large household in Tennessee.

Both Adeline Blanchard Tyler and Sallie Chapman Gordon Law took on managerial roles in small hospitals during the early days of the war. The quality of their early work is attested to by the significant roles they each played in larger hospitals later in their careers. At Chester Hospital, Tyler took charge of the care of almost a thousand patients. And the Southern Mothers' Hospital met with such success under Law's management that it had to take over larger quarters; eventually, it provided care for more than two thousand men. Both women excelled in their roles as organizers, leaders, and nurses. They each ignored the social stricture that confined women to the home during the national crisis and instead rendered their services as nurses within male-dominated military and medical structures. Both women were honored for their contributions to the care of soldiers: Tyler with a citation from the Massachusetts Legislature, and Law with a parade of troops.

A final parallel between these two women can be seen in their experience of caring for soldiers from the opposing side. Although each woman was loyal to her own cause during the war, philosophical differences did not hinder either from rendering humanitarian care to those in need. In this fashion, Adeline Blanchard Tyler and Sallie Chapman Gordon Law helped to establish nursing as a caring force that transcended political boundaries.[43]

Thus the first nurses of the Civil War contributed much more than their care for the soldiers. They defied society's limitations that would confine them to "a woman's sphere." These two women left their homes and served their respective causes as best they could. Tyler and Law did not rely on tradition to dictate their actions, but instead contributed to the war effort, to the beginnings of organized nursing, and to the fabric of the postwar society.

Quincealea Brunk, PhD, RN, CCRN
The University of Alabama School of Nursing
The University of Alabama at Birmingham
1701 8th Avenue South
Birmingham, Ala. 35294-1210
Phone: (205) 934-6583
Fax: (205) 934-1894

Acknowledgments

A special acknowledgment is made to Dr. Eleanor L. M. Crowder and Dr. Diane K. Kjervik for their support of the dissertation from which this article was taken.

Notes

1. Nancy F. Cott, *The Grounding of Modern Feminism* (New Haven, Conn.: Yale University Press, 1987). See also Catharine Clinton, *The Other Civil War* (New York: Hill and Wang, 1984); James P. Lowis, "The Roots of Feminism: A Review Essay," *Civil War History* 17, no. 2 (June 1971): 162–70.

2. Bonnie Bullough and Vern Bullough, "The Origins of Modern American Nursing: The Civil War Era," *Nursing Forum* 11, no. 2 (1963): 12–27; Philip A. Kalisch and Beatrice J. Kalisch, "Untrained but Undaunted: The Women Nurses of the Blue and the Gray," *Nursing Forum* 15, no. 1 (1976): 4–33; Myrtle P. Matejski,

"Ladies' Aid Societies and the Nurses of Lincoln's Army," *Journal of Nursing History* 1, no. 2 (April 1986): 35–51; Isabel Quattlebaum, "Twelve Women in the First Days of the Confederacy," *Civil War History* 7, no. 4 (December 1961): 370–87.

3. Edward T. James, Janet Wilson James, and Paul S. Boyer, eds., "Adeline Blanchard Tyler," *Notable American Women 1670–1950* (Cambridge, Mass.: Harvard University Press, Belknap Press, 1971), 3:491; "Adeline Blanchard Tyler," Dielman-Hayward file, Maryland Historical Society, Baltimore.

4. Judith Robinson, *Ensign on a Hill. The Story of the Church Home and Hospital and its School of Nursing 1854–1954* (Baltimore, Md.: Church Home and Hospital, 1954), 11–17.

5. Robinson, 23–24.

6. Robinson, 27.

7. E. B. Long, *The Civil War Day by Day: An Almanac 1861–1865* (New York: Da Capo Press, 1971), 62–63.

8. Alexander Fulton, handwritten account of the events related to Tyler on 19 April 1861, Adeline Blanchard Tyler Collection, Maryland Historical Society, Baltimore; a manuscript labeled "Hospital Work—Baltimore Chester Anapolis," written by Tyler's sister, also in the Adeline Blanchard Tyler Collection, Maryland Historical Society, Baltimore (hereafter cited as ABT); and Robinson, 28.

9. Fulton, 10, ABT.

10. Julia C. Stimson and Ethel C. S. Thompson, "Women Nurses With the Union Forces During the Civil War," Part I *Military Surgeon* 62 (January 1928): 3.

11. "Hospital Work," ABT.

12. "Hospital Work," ABT.

13. "Hospital Work," ABT, 126.

14. Copy of letter from Bishop Whittingham, Baltimore, to Rev. Hammond, Chaplain Chester Hospital, 30 August 1862, contained in "Hospital Work," ABT.

15. Tyler, New York, to Bishop Whittingham, Baltimore, 3 September 1862, ABT.

16. Tyler, New York, to her sister, 12 September 1862, ABT.

17. Tyler, Chester Hospital, to her sister, 3 October 1862, ABT.

18. "Hospital Work," 133–35, ABT.

19. Diary entry for 8 July 1863 as copied in "Hospital Work," 135–37, ABT.

20. Diary entry as copied in "Hospital Work," ABT.

21. Diary entry as copied in "Hospital Work," 138, ABT.

22. Tyler, Annapolis, to her sister, 15 December 1863, contained in "Hospital Work," ABT.

23. Tyler, Naval School Hospital, Annapolis, to her sister, 27 February 1863, copied in "Hospital Work," ABT.

24. James, James, and Boyer, 3:491.

25. Mrs. S[allie] C[hapman] Law, *Reminiscences of the War of the Sixties between the North and South* (Memphis, Tenn.: Memphis Press, 1892), 3–4.

26. Allen Johnson and Dumas Malone, eds., "Sallie Chapman Gordon Law," *Dictionary of American Biography* (New York: Charles Scribner's Sons, 1929), 6:42–43; "Sallie Chapman (Gordon) Law," *The National Cyclopedia of American Biography* (New York: James T. White and Co., 1893), 25:347–48.

27. Law, 4; *National Cyclopedia,* 25:348.

28. *National Cyclopedia,* 25:348; Law, 4–5.

29. This would date Law's presence in Columbus for 3 and 4 September 1861. See E. B. Long, 114–15.

30. Law, 6–7.

31. Law, 7.

32. Law, 8.

33. According to Long, 221–23, the defense and surrender of Memphis, and its subsequent occupation by Union troops, occurred quickly—between 2 and 7 June 1862. Thus, the estimated closing of the Southern Mothers' Hospital was near this period of time. See also *National Cyclopedia,* 25:348.

34. Law, 8–9.

35. Law, 9.

36. Law, 11.

37. Law, 14.

38. *National Cyclopedia,* 25:348; "A Mother of the Confederacy," *Southern Historical Society Papers* 22 (July 1894): 63–64.

39. Law, 16.

40. *National Cyclopedia,* 25:348; *Dictionary of American Biography,* 6:43. After the war, Southern Mothers' Society became Southern Mothers' Association.

41. Law, 16.

42. "A Mother of the Confederacy," 64; *National Cyclopedia,* 25:348; *Dictionary of American Biography,* 6:43.

43. The International Red Cross was founded in Europe in 1869 but did not receive ratification in the United States until 1882. Conventions regarding the humane treatment of prisoners were not in operation in the United States until the twentieth century. Thus, the nurses of the Civil War set a precedent in their humane treatment of soldiers from the opposing side.

The Educational and Philosophical Influences on Florence Nightingale, An Enlightened Conductor

Victoria E. Slater
College of Nursing
University of Tennessee, Knoxville

I began this research under the assumption that Florence Nightingale was ahead of her time and that her thinking was holistic. However, a review of nursing literature, a close look at Florence Nightingale's biographies, and a study of the cultural influences of her day led me to realize that she was, indeed, a woman of her time. Her words and deeds reflected the prevailing philosophical beliefs concerning the leaders of society, the assigned role of women, and the accepted assumptions that the mind and body were separate, unintegrated entities.

To put Nightingale's life in perspective, it is necessary to investigate the life and education of the average upper-class English woman of the early 1800s. One must understand the influence of Rousseau's and Descartes's philosophies as well as appreciate the profound changes in English society wrought by the Industrial Revolution. During such study, an image gradually emerges of how upper-class English women in the second quarter of the nineteenth century were taught to view themselves. Only then can the body of literature written about Florence Nightingale be reanalyzed, revealing how the social and philosophical influences of her time guided her actions and shored up her determination.

Two themes emerged from this research. The first was the importance of the classical education given Nightingale by her father. Of equal significance was the role of women in Victorian England during the Industrial Revolution. The tension between the two types of education she received gave rise to the Florence Nightingale who changed the lives of British soldiers and nursing forever.

Nursing History Review 2 (1994): 137–152.

Her Father's Influence: A Philosophical Education

The Nightingale family ignored the prevailing upper-class English custom of offering little or no education to female children. William Nightingale and his wife had two daughters: Florence, born in 1820, and Parthenope, born in 1819. When the time came for their education, Nightingale, a classically educated gentleman, chose to give them a broad education at home, including the study of philosophy, languages (Greek, Latin, French, and Italian), mathematics, science, and astronomy. Although the classics were ordinarily reserved for men, William Nightingale was determined to teach his daughters well. Young Florence was a quick and eager scholar who matched her father's interests and discussed with him a wide range of ideas. Her sister, however, was less interested in scholarship; she focused instead on her mother's activities and other pursuits deemed appropriate for women of the day. Florence, therefore, spent much of her time in the company of her father and absorbed the best of his world; it is not too farfetched to surmise that she was "her father's darling."[1] The foundation for her life's work was being set into place as she sat at her father's feet.

During the course of his daughters' education, Nightingale apparently put more emphasis on the study of philosophy than on any other discipline. Four philosophers' teachings were to become cornerstones of Florence Nightingale's personal identity, bringing within her a confluence of her concept of self, the real world and its needs, and the duty to the truth as she perceived it. The first of the philosophers she studied was Descartes.

René Descartes

In 1643 the French philosopher René Descartes, struggling to understand consciousness, concluded with his famous dictum, *Cogito, ergo sum,* "I think, therefore I am." Unfortunately for twentieth-century thinkers trying to understand Descartes and the ramifications of his philosophy, that phrase does not bring to our minds the same images as it did to Descartes and his nineteenth-century students. The vision he put forth was that "the world of reality is divided into two ultimate and irreducible elements," two discrete substances: mind (soul) and matter.[2] All things that were material in nature obeyed mechanical and mathematical laws and were, in fact, machines. Animals, plants, people, and the planet earth were machines; only the soul and God were not.

Superimposed on some machines was the mind, or soul, a separate entity from the machine. God, who created the universe, had created his matter, which included all bodily functions and movements, to obey mechanical principles. Some of that matter he had given souls, thereby forming human beings. Animals and some people—those who had not been given minds, for example—were considered soulless machines. The debate over whether women had souls, seen in the light of Descartes's philosophy, centered on whether women could be considered to be like machines, and thus animals, or whether they were in fact human. If they were human, were they as completely human as men?

Much of Florence Nightingale's reading pertained to this debate and its corollary: Should women be educated, and, if so, how? The question was considered by three authors: Plato, Jean-Jacques Rousseau, and Dugald Stewart.

Plato

Plato's views of the role and education of women are given in *The Republic,* a major work in which he advances his vision of the Just State.[3] Plato believed that women as a class were inferior to men—an understandable conclusion considering that during the fourth and fifth centuries B.C., women in Athens were little more than slaves.[4] Plato argued, however, that "the present status of women is a perversion of nature and a waste of the resources of half the population."[5] He believed that women and men should be educated equally for the highest functions of the state. Although he did not expect that many women would be capable of handling the best education, he acknowledged that there would be exceptions. The young Florence no doubt knew she must be an exception.

Plato made two primary assumptions regarding human nature. The first proposed that each person is born with a specific aptitude, or talent, for one task more than for others; this talent is innate but must be developed through education. Plato believed that throughout the state all the different aptitudes necessary for its proper functioning are available, but that within one person there is a primary aptitude for only one task.[6] Plato, however, did not believe that sex determined one's nature. Although he acknowledged that women were different from men, that difference did not affect the person's innate nature.[7]

Plato's second assumption further clarifies his view of human nature. He believed that a division of labor was needed for the good of the state. This division took the form of three basic roles: artisan, auxiliary, and ruler. Each person's innate aptitude defined the one category into which he or she fit. Members of the artisan class were born to perform all of the city's physical maintenance. Soldiers, who were of the auxiliary class, were responsible for the city's defense. The members of these two classes were urged to be moderate in their activities and were believed to be "dominated by either appetite or spirit, neither of which are said to be uniquely human traits."[8] Guardians of the Just State, who came from two classes, auxiliary and ruler, were a special category of citizens, the "philosopher-kings." Only their functions were "noble and worth pursuing for their own sake," rather than solely for the functioning of the city.[9] Their work was philosophic wisdom, from which would emerge justice for the city and its citizens. To be free to pursue intellectual and philosophical interests, from which would emerge justice, guardians needed to be free of practical concerns, such as "responsibility and trouble of caring for children."[10] These duties were relegated to the artisan and auxiliary classes.

Where did this leave women? Actually, in two places. Plato believed that, in general, women should be held in common, like other property.[11] However, a few women would be guardians and they, too, should be freed from daily domestic and parental time-consuming tasks and be responsible for the honor of the city.[12]

Plato defined traits for the three classes. Of significance for Nightingale were the characteristics of guardians; they would be

> brave and high-spirited, because a high spirit makes the soul fearless. They must love wisdom. If they are to be rulers, moreover, they must be rational thinkers, able not only to distinguish the Good by their reason but to argue their case according to reality rather than opinions, while surviving refutations of it. The capacity for rational thought is not enough; reason must rule the individuals who rule.[13]

Jean-Jacques Rousseau

Jean-Jacques Rousseau discussed the education of women in his 1762 treatise *Emile*. Although *Emile* was published sixty years before Nightingale was born, Rousseau's concept of the role of women permeated Victorian culture and contributed to that society's expectations for upper-class women. Rousseau accepted Descartes's view that mind and matter were separate entities and believed that the female machine had, in fact, been given less soul, less mind, than the male machine. Therefore, Rousseau argued, the female machine was designed for the male machine. He wrote that men should be active and strong with power and will; women, however, should be passive and weak with little power of resistance. Rousseau believed that men and women, therefore, should have different educations.

> Does it follow that [women] ought to be brought up in complete ignorance, and restricted solely to the duties of the household? No. . . . They ought to learn multitudes of things, but only those which it becomes them to know. . . . Thus the whole education of women ought to be relative to man. To please them, to be useful to them, to make themselves loved and honored by them . . . and to make life agreeable and sweet to them—these are the duties of women at all times, and what should be taught them from their infancy. . . . She must therefore make a profound study of the mind of man, not the mind of man in general, through abstraction, but the mind of the men who surround her, the mind of the men to whom she is subject, either by law or by opinion. She must learn to penetrate their feelings through their conversation, their actions, their looks, and their gestures.
>
> A woman of wit is the scourge of her husband, her children, her friends, her servants, of everybody. . . . Her dignity is leading a retired life; her glory is in the esteem of her husband; her pleasures are in the happiness of her family.[14]

Dugald Stewart

Sir Edward Cook's *Life of Florence Nightingale,* the only biography authorized by the Nightingale family, records that Florence Nightingale "analyzed Dugald Stewart's *Elements of the Philosophy of the Human Mind.*"[15] Dugald Stewart taught moral philosophy at the University of Edinburgh and first published his book in 1792, thereafter updating it in 1814 and 1842. In the first part of the book, Stewart agrees with Descartes's division of mind and matter and with the premise that people of different natures should be educated differently. He then leaps to a discussion of how physics and philosophy are similar: Physics, he writes, seeks to discover the laws and principles by which matter works; philosophy seeks to discover the laws and principles by which mind works. Physics has made more progress, according to Stewart, because the results are more obvious. He argues that this does not mean, however, that one cannot discover the principles by which the mind works.

Stewart goes on to explain principles of the mind, offering a formula for the proper educational approach for people of different natures. The following quotations echo Plato's argument that people are given inherent gifts and that education should be designed to enhance these gifts. Stewart's writings also evoke images of Plato's guardians and their responsibilities: Stewart suggests that "enlightened conductors" write down the practical rules they learn by experience so that others may benefit from their insights.

> The most essential objects of education are . . . to cultivate all the various principles of our nature, both speculative [mind] and active [body], in

> such a manner as to bring them to the greatest perfection of which they are susceptible.[16]
>
> Surely the great aim of an enlightened and benevolent philosophy, is not to rear a small number of individuals, who may be regarded as prodigies in an ignorant and admiring age, but to diffuse, as widely as possible, that degree of cultivation which may enable the bulk of a people to possess all the intellectual and moral improvement of which their nature is susceptible.[17]
>
> If the multitude must be led, it is of consequence, surely, that it should be led by enlightened conductors; by men who are able to distinguish truth from error.[18]
>
> In the case of individuals, who have no other guide to direct them in their inquiries than their own natural sagacity, much time and ingenuity must inevitably be thrown away. . . . The misfortune is . . . that . . . the aids which the understanding derives from experience, are seldom recorded in writing. . . . If the more important practical rules . . . were diligently preserved, each generation would be placed in circumstances more favorable to invention than the preceding; and the progress of knowledge, instead of cramping original genius, would assist and direct its exertions.[19]

Descartes and Rousseau prescribed narrow boundaries for women, especially for one with so broad a mind as Florence Nightingale. Stewart and Plato, however, provided Nightingale with an image of the guardian, an enlightened conductor, which was a role open to only a few men and fewer women. Many of Nightingale's actions in her career reflect tenets outlined by Stewart, as well as the views of Plato and Descartes on the dual nature of people. Primarily, her actions reflect Stewart's and Plato's belief of the elite's responsibilities to society.

Her Mother's Influence: An Upper-Class Victorian Lady

Women in Victorian England

Nightingale's times were tumultuous. Victorian England has been described as a time of a "violently contrasted, rapidly changing life," which began "with gentlemen fighting duels . . . [and ended] with gentlemen playing golf."[20] Nightingale was born seventeen years before Victoria came to rule as queen, a reign that some believe marked the division between the ancient and modern worlds.[21] Nightingale's early childhood and education took place, by that estimation, in the ancient world.

In the "ancient" world, the lady in rural England occupied a clearly marked role, with prescribed behaviors and expectations; women who worked were looked down upon. The Industrial Revolution began in the mid-1700s, and by the early 1800s, the hands of a few held the majority of wealth. Because the husband provided all income, the role of the upper-class woman was to symbolize the wealth of the husband.[22] Women were grouped along with children and idiots, and when they married their property became their husband's. For example, in a will written in the early 1800s, a generous husband "left to Mathilde, his beloved wife, the silver candlesticks which her loving father gave to her as a wedding-present."[23] Any children the couple had belonged to the husband; divorce was virtually impossible.[24] A woman's only purpose was to be a wife and mother. Her primary objective was to get married. As Rousseau wrote, a woman's object was to please the man she married.

The classical education that Florence Nightingale, as a female in Victorian England, received from her father was "just for fun"; she was never expected to use it.[25] Instead, her mother offered the more important learning. Nightingale described her mother as a woman of genius: "She has the genius of order . . . the genius to organize a parish, to form society."[26] Nightingale learned to run a household, with all of its varied tasks, and to supervise servants and look after their welfare. She also learned the accomplishments expected of a young Victorian lady—needlework, singing, playing the piano, drawing, flower arranging, dancing, congenial conversation—all of which contributed to her primary responsibility as a female to provide a harmonious home for her family, particularly for the men in her circle. An ancillary role, but an important one, was visiting the tenants who resided on her father's lands and seeing to their welfare. "Poor-peopling," Nightingale called it.[27]

Nightingale's social life followed closely the social season. From April to July and from October to Christmas the family was in London. The London social season in turn coincided with Parliamentary sessions, and much of the social conversation would surround the debates and issues before Parliament and the current political gossip.[28] This may have been a crucial training ground for Nightingale's expertise in the art of influencing powerful men. The rest of the year the Nightingale family traveled between the two family homes, visiting, or being visited by, some of their numerous relatives.

An Unhappy Florence Nightingale

Florence Nightingale began to feel a smoldering dissatisfaction with the restricted life of women.[29] As a young lady she wrote:

> A profession, a trade, a necessary occupation, something to fill and employ all my faculties, I have always felt essential to me, I have always longed for, consciously or not. . . . The first thought I can remember, and the last, was nursing work. . . . My God! What is to become of me?[30]

Another time she wrote:

> Why, oh, my God, cannot I be satisfied with the life that satisfies so many people? Why am I starving, desperate, diseased upon it? . . . Oh, how I have longed for a trial to give me food, to be something real. A nourishing life—that is the happiness, whatever it be. A starving life, that is the real trial. My God, what am I to do? Teach me, tell me.[31]

And at the age of twenty-six she wrote:

> Very few people lead such an impoverishing and confusing and weakening life as the women of the richer classes. . . . We do the best we can to train our women to an idle, superficial life; we teach them music and drawing, languages and poor peopling—"resources" as they're called, and we hope if they don't marry they will at least be quiet.[32]

She also wrote that both men and women see women "as a great curiosity—a peculiar strange race, like the Aztecs; or rather like Dr. Howe's Idiots, whom, after the 'unremitting exertions of two years,' he 'actually taught to eat with a spoon.'"[33]

Escape from such rigid and repressive society was imperative for this woman who could "eat with many spoons." Her bitterness and anger resound through her writings. Her mother and sister did not understand her dissatisfaction with the role of a Victorian lady, and her father did not understand why she was not content with private studies. He thought her restlessness would pass when she got married.[34] Nightingale, however, had other ideas about marriage. She wrote: "Some few sacrifice marriage, because they sacrifice all other life if they accept that."[35] In 1846 she wrote: "I think He [Providence] has as clearly marked out some to be single women as He has others to be wives, and has organized them accordingly for their vocation."[36] Rejecting marriage, she looked for other studies and chose mathematics. Her father, however, refused to hire her a tutor. After all, mathematics were of no use to a married woman.[37]

One activity that was open to her was charitable work. Yet even for this noble work, there were strict Victorian rules. One could offer sympathy and small gifts, but concrete action was not permitted.[38] In her early twenties, Nightingale broke out of her proper boundaries and began to visit the cottages and tenants on the estates of her family and of other relatives. What she found appalled her. The tenant families lived in crowded, damp, filthy, poorly ventilated cottages, averaging ten feet square. There was no easy way for them to wash themselves or their clothing. During inclement weather, if an effort were made to wash clothing, such as diapers, or if clothing got wet, the garments had to be hung indoors. The next morning, these same clothes would be put on wet because there was no room and little or no heat for them to dry thoroughly. Needless to say, illness was common.[39]

Nightingale broke convention by doing more than expressing sympathy and making gifts of food and flowers. She began doing small nursing tasks. As she became more skilled, she realized she needed training, and so at twenty-four years of age, she requested permission to study nursing. Her mother and sister became hysterical; her father called her "spoiled" and "ungrateful." Nightingale backed down. For the next seven years, she went in and out of depressions, all the while secretly studying government reports about social conditions and fledgling efforts at reform. By the time she was thirty, she was an expert on government social statistics, and her friend, Sidney Herbert, who was Secretary to the Admiralty, began seeking her opinion.[40]

The turning point for her family was their realization that Nightingale's continuing depression was serious; they became concerned for her stability. Her desire to become a nurse had not passed; it had become more persistent. In 1851, after many years of requesting permission and being refused, she informed her family that, despite their objections, she was going to Germany to train at the Institution of Deaconesses at Kaiserswerth. They finally relented, asking, however, that she tell no one where she was going. Friends were told that Nightingale was going to a spa at Carlsbad for a three-month rest.

When Nightingale returned to England filled with plans to train in a large London hospital, she found that her father had fallen ill. Soon after she herself came down with measles. During a trip the two took to recuperate, Nightingale must have been both persuasive and an attentive caregiver.[41] When they returned from their trip, her father informed his family of his support for Nightingale's goals. Two years later, in 1853, she accepted her first position as the unpaid superintendent of the Institution for the Care of Sick Gentlewomen, otherwise known as the Harley Street Nursing Home. Her father granted her an allowance, and she established herself independently in London.[42]

The Effect of Her Philosophical and Practical Educations

What would have made a lovely, accomplished Victorian country lady spend years secretly studying something so laborious as governmental reports on social conditions? What would make her persist in her desire to train for work that only the lowliest women and nuns did? The answer to these questions may lie in the works of Plato and Stewart.

When Nightingale wrote "Why . . . cannot I be satisfied with the life that satisfies so many people?," she may have been asking if she had been given more "mind" than most women.[43] Was she more like a man than a woman in her mental nature? There is, indeed, some evidence that she may have believed so. In her diary she wrote, as if to her mother;

> Why, my dear, you don't suppose that with my "talents" and my "European reputation" and my "beautiful letters," and all that, I'm going to stay dangling about my mother's drawing-room all my life! I shall go and look out for work, to be sure. You must look upon me as your son.[44]

In her later life, she described herself as a "man of action" or a "man of business."[45]

An Enlightened Conductor

When she looked at her life in the light of Plato's and Stewart's writings, Nightingale may have come to see herself as one of Plato's guardians. She was one of the elite, one of Stewart's enlightened conductors. This was her nature, her inherent gift, and her education was appropriate for one who was to lead the multitudes.

A very religious person, Nightingale felt she had a call from God.[46] In 1852 she wrote that God called her to be a savior, and she defined savior as "one who saves from error." She believed that "the world never seems to make much progress except by Saviors."[47] Once she had decided how that call was to be manifested, her role as a guardian became more clear: She was to open nursing to respectable women. In 1854, while at the Harley Street Nursing Home, she outlined plans for training farmers' daughters as nurses.[48]

The Dual Nature of the Human

Nightingale's view of the body and mind as separate entities and her consideration of how the "flesh and spirit" fit into the role of nursing as she understood it can be seen in her daily logs from Harley Street, in letters written during that time, and in her actions in the Crimea. She followed Stewart's admonitions carefully, being concerned with both body and mind. In 1854, for example, she wrote that one patient who had been discharged from Harley Street was "physically in the same state morally worse."[49] While at Harley Street she subscribed for the patients, at her own expense, to the London *Times,* but then wrote:

> A Hospital is good for the seriously ill alone—otherwise it becomes a lodging-house where the nervous become more nervous, the foolish more foolish, the idle & selfish more selfish & idle. For two of the elements essential to a Hospital are want of occupation & directing the attention to bodily health.[50]

She believed that only those patients who were unable to help themselves or who were dying needed nursing. Her famous saying, "What nursing has to do . . . is to put the patient in the best condition for nature to act upon him," meant that nurses should put the human machine in optimal condition for the machine of nature to act upon it.[51]

In 1854, the Crimean War sidelined Nightingale's plan to train nurses. It also served to clarify for her her view of nursing and of her own role as a guardian of the state. She was to be the guardian of the British soldier.

As a guardian in the Crimea, Nightingale's first significant change to standard procedure was her approach to the material nature of the human machine, the body. The "really sick" patients received care similar to that given today: "watching, giving medication under doctors' orders, feeding under doctors' orders, and washing patients and bed linen."[52] However, she also called upon her mother's training in housekeeping skills and saw that the building and water supply were cleaned and that the open privys were closed. Her mother's training probably prepared Nightingale for the task of cleaning the Scutari Barracks and guided her in the supervision of the nurses and orderlies.

Her second major effort in the Crimea was to intervene with the mental nature of the human. By doing so she refuted Descartes's view of men as mechanical animals without minds. Rather, she treated the soldiers as if they were humans with souls. As Stewart recommended, education should "cultivate all the various principles of our nature."[53] Nightingale began classes, provided books and periodicals, encouraged the men to write their families, and provided paper and stamps. She established a cafe to provide an alternative to the canteens, where the primary refreshment was alcohol. She persuaded men to send their pay home and established a banking system to enable them to do so.[54]

She described the bank in a letter written to General Sir Howard Douglas from Scutari Barracks in January 1856. In her usual style, Nightingale praised the person to whom the letter was addressed.

> I feel more encouraged by the support & confidence of those who, like you, have labored all their lives for the benefit of the soldiers so wisely & so successfully, than by any feeling of my own success. . . . I have done my little utmost to serve as a Savings Bank & transmitter of money home for the men & have exercised the latter office at the rate of 1,000 pounds per month in small sums in this Depot alone- . . . I assure you that I will do all in my power to promote the Savings Banks . . . no one, not even yourself, has felt more deeply than I have the cruel injury to the soldier's moral character in the Crimea, consequent upon his being driven into drink by plenty of money & nothing to do with it.[55]

Rousseau's and Stewart's Influences

I believe Nightingale accomplished much of what she did by going back to her study of Rousseau. She felt encouraged to "make a profound study of the mind of man," in particular the minds of the men who surrounded her. She had been urged to "penetrate their feelings through their conversation, their actions, their looks, and their gestures."[56] Her years as a participant in British social circles gave her the opportunity to observe the men around her and learn to "penetrate their feelings." In an 1853 letter to her father, from her position as superintendent of the Upper Harley Street Nursing Home, she described the effect of her study.

> When I entered into service here, I determined that, happen what would, I *never* would intrigue among the Com'tee. Now I perceive that I do all my business by intrigue. I propose in private to A, B, or C the resolution I think A, B, or C most capable of carrying in Com'tee, & then leave it to them—& I always win.[57]

In a letter from the Crimea to Sidney Herbert, she described her first attempts to bathe the soldiers and the problems she was having in meeting their needs. She closed with a note of caution: "All the above is written in obedience to your *private* instructions. Do not let me appear as a Gov't spy here which would destroy all my usefulness."[58]

Stewart urged that the important practical rules that the enlightened learn from their own experience be written down. Nightingale, the guardian of the British soldier, did so. Her results can be seen in four of her treatises: *Notes on Matters Affecting the Health, Efficiency, and Hospital Administration of the British Army* (1858), *Subsidiary Notes as to the Introduction of Female Nursing into Military Hospitals (1858), Notes on Hospitals* (1859), and *Notes on Nursing* (1860). The first three are filled with recommendations formulated through her studies of government reports and tours of hospitals in England and Europe, as well as from her experiences in the Crimea. The third, in particular, suggests an approach to the organization and design of hospitals and the administration and support of female nurses.[59]

Notes on Nursing was written not for nurses but for all women who were responsible for caring for their own families. It was to become the first nursing textbook, however, and many of its revolutionary concepts are standard hygienic practices today.[60] As Stewart envisioned, her approach toward "diligently [preserving] . . . the more important practical rules" furthered the "progress of knowledge."[61]

Conclusion

Florence Nightingale put all of her education to good use. Her studies of the classics and the philosophers set before her a model of the enlightened conductor, the leader of the multitudes, the savior, the guardian of the Just State. Her standing as a member of the social elite and as a Victorian country lady who was expected to fulfill the woman's role portrayed by Rousseau gave her both the theoretical and the practical wherewithal to influence the powerful men through whom she had to work. Stewart's *Elements of the Philosophy of the Human Mind* gave her guidance and direction for caring for the mental aspect of the human animal. The principles of cleanliness and organization she learned from her mother led the way to the changes in sanitation that were responsible for the extraordinary drop in mortality rates in the Crimea. Although Nightingale was a creature of Victorian England, she was able to use the education and training available to her to "guide the multitudes" and begin a new work. She was able to serve as guardian for the British soldier, which contributed to opening the vocation of nursing to respectable women.

Victoria E. Slater, MSN, RN
Doctoral Candidate
College of Nursing
University of Tennessee, Knoxville

2712 Trelawny Drive
Clarksville, Tenn. 37043
Phone: (615) 358-9410

Acknowledgments

The author acknowledges the guidance of Dr. Clinton Allison of the University of Tennessee, Knoxville, Department of Curriculum and Instruction, and the assistance of Charlotte Marshall and Karen Johnson, whose editorial abilities and literary bents gave the finishing touches to this work.

Notes

1. Sir Edward Cook, *The Life of Florence Nightingale* (New York and London: Macmillan, 1942), 13.
2. Amaury de Riencourt, *Sex and Power in History* (New York: David McKay, 1974), 264.
3. Jane Roland Martin, *Reclaiming A Conversation: The Ideal of the Educated Woman* (New Haven, Conn.: Yale University Press, 1985), 12.
4. Lynda L. Lange, "The Function of Equal Education in Plato's Republic and Laws," in *The Sexism of Social and Political Theory: Women and Reproduction from Plato to Nietzsche,* ed. Lorenne M. G. Clark and Lynda Lange (Toronto: University of Toronto Press, 1979), 2.
5. Rosemary Agonito, *History of Ideas on Woman: A Source Book* (New York: Capricorn Books, 1977), 23.
6. Martin, 13.
7. Ibid., 14.
8. Lange, 6.
9. Ibid.
10. Ibid., 8.
11. Ibid., 9.
12. Martin, 15.
13. Ibid., 28.
14. Jean-Jacques Rousseau, "Emile," in *Women from the Greeks to the French Revolution,* ed. Susan G. Bell (Belmont: Wadsworth, 1973), 263–66.
15. Cook, 13.
16. Dugald Stewart, *Elements of the Philosophy of the Human Mind* (Boston, Mass.: James Munroe and Company, 1842), 20.
17. Stewart, 24.
18. Ibid., 26.
19. Ibid., 36.
20. Duncan Crow, *The Victorian Woman* (London: George Allen and Unwin, Ltd., 1971), 11–12.
21. Ibid., 12–13.
22. Ibid., 45–47.
23. Margaret Goldsmith, *Seven Women Against the World* (London: Wethuen and Co., 1976), 223.

24. Crow, 146–47.

25. Margaret Forster, *Significant Sisters: The Grassroots of Active Feminism 1839–1939* (New York: Alfred A. Knopf, 1985), 98.

26. Cook, 105.

27. Crow, 62.

28. Ibid., 34.

29. Forster, 97.

30. Cook, 106.

31. Vera Brittain, *Lady into Woman: A History of Women from Victoria to Elizabeth II* (New York: Macmillan, 1953), 27.

32. Crow, 42.

33. Evelyn L. Pugh, "Florence Nightingale and J. S. Mill Debate Women's Rights," *Journal of British Studies* 21 (Spring 1982): 123.

34. Forster, 100.

35. Brittain, 174.

36. Cook, 100.

37. Pamela Horn, *Victorian Countrywomen* (Cambridge, Mass.: Basil Blackwell, 1991), 59.

38. Crow, 62–63.

39. Ibid., 90–92.

40. Forster, 101–3.

41. Cook, 118.

42. Sylvia Strauss, "Florence Nightingale and the Bonds of Sisterhood," in *The Sister Bond: A Feminist View of a Timeless Connection,* ed. Toni A. H. McNaron (New York: Pergamon, 1985), 77.

43. Brittain, 27.

44. Cook, 122.

45. Bonnie S. Anderson and Judith P. Zinsser, *A History of Their Own: Women in Europe from Prehistory to the Present* (New York: Harper and Row, 1988), 2:168.

46. Cecil Woodham-Smith, *Florence Nightingale: 1820–1910* (New York: McGraw-Hill, Inc., 1951), 12.

47. Joann G. Widerquist, "The Spirituality of Florence Nightingale," *Nursing Research* 41, no. 1 (January/February 1992): 52.

48. Pam Brown, *Florence Nightingale* (Watford: Exley, 1988), 23.

49. Florence Nightingale, *Florence Nightingale at Harley Street: Her Reports to the Governors of Her Nursing Home 1953–4,* ed. Sir Harry Verney (London: J. M. Dent and Sons, 1970), 13.

50. Nightingale, *Harley Street,* 6, 15.

51. Florence Nightingale, "Notes on Nursing: What It Is and What It Is Not," in *Selected Writings of Florence Nightingale,* ed. L. R. Seymer (New York: MacMillan, 1954), 214.

52. Francis Barrymore Smith, *Florence Nightingale: Reputation and Power,* (London: Croom Helm, 1982), 35.

53. Stewart, 20.

54. Sarah A. Tooley, *The Life of Florence Nightingale* (London: Cassel and Company, Ltd., 1910), 231–32.

55. Florence Nightingale, *Letters of Florence Nightingale in the History of Nursing Archive, Special Collections, Boston University Libraries,* ed. Lois A. Monteiro (Boston, Mass.: Boston University, 1974), 4.

56. Rousseau, 266.

57. Florence Nightingale, *Ever Yours, Florence Nightingale: Selected Letters,* ed. Martha Vicinus and Bea Nergaard (Cambridge, Mass.: Harvard University Press, 1990), 74–75.

58. Nightingale, *Ever Yours,* 88–89.

59. Nightingale, *Notes on Nursing,* 1–122.

60. Woodham-Smith, 228.

61. Stewart, 36.

Nursing Uniforms: Romantic Idea, Functional Attire, or Instrument of Social Change?

Irene Schuessler Poplin
Division of Nursing
Midwestern State University

The history of modern secular nursing uniforms, which identify a female wearer as belonging to the nursing profession, originated with Theodor and Friedericke Fliedner, who in 1836 founded the Kaiserswerth Deaconess Institute's Nurse Training School.[1] The Fliedners had a vision that they hoped to translate into a practical reality. They saw standard uniform attire as fundamental to the new, modern nursing occupation because the nurse had to have a respectable and competent outward appearance, both as an individual and as a member of a respected occupational group.[2] Their views differed from conceptions of nursing held by Florence Nightingale and her contemporaries, for whom uniforms were not an issue but a mere practical matter. But, in early nineteenth-century Prussia, later to become Germany, where the Fliedners labored to gain recognition and social respectability for the new nursing, attire was a matter of vital importance. Without uniforms signaling respectability in a very class-structured, rigidly controlled, authoritarian society, nursing could not have succeeded. Respectable women could not have overcome the loathsome reputation associated with the "derelicts" hired to do hospital nursing. As it was, nurses not only became recognizable by their dress, but their uniform clothing came to symbolize caring, professional competence, and, above all, unquestionable moral character. Distinguished by their uniform dress, these unmarried women engaged in nursing the public. The uniform signified that they could be trusted to conduct themselves according to narrowly defined social boundaries—in short, to adhere to paternalistic mores.

Nursing History Review 2 (1994): 153–167.

Image Building

According to historian Susan Reverby, character, above all else, differentiated the trained Nightingale nurse from her untrained predecessors. In this, "behavior and demeanor" as much as skill became "the hallmark of the trained nurse."[3] Although important to Nightingale's system, these characteristics were even more elemental to Theodor Fliedner's earlier vision of nursing. Fully aware that his idea of making proper women employable outside the home would be resisted because it proposed to reform important traditional customs, and knowing that success hinged on overcoming strong opposition to his viewpoints, he set out to create a powerful, public image of the new female occupation.[4] To this end he invented the nursing uniform.

Although Friedericke Fliedner, as first matron, contributed to the implementation of a uniform policy, it was her husband who conceived the idea. Theodor Fliedner was a Lutheran minister compelled by a mission to establish nursing in Protestant Prussia equal to, but preferably better than, that provided by Catholic religious women in the Catholic regions of Germany. In so doing, he hoped to found nursing as a reputable occupation for honorable, single, Protestant women who otherwise had no means for working outside the home.[5] Nursing was to be organized as a Protestant Christian order: its members would serve Christ by giving care as deaconess nurses.[6] As an association, the order would provide social and occupational status; job, illness, and retirement security; and the opportunity for selfless Christian work for its members. In Protestant Prussia, especially for populations of the newly pauperized industrial working class, nurses would ensure dedicated, competent care in hospitals and the community.[7] This dual purpose of occupational dignity for its members and Christian social service for the community had to be conveyed through the image of the dress.

Fliedner, his first wife Friedericke, and after Friedericke's death in 1848, his second wife Caroline attached great importance to dress because it conveyed role and status and differentiated Kaiserswerth nurses from the common, disreputable attendants hired to nurse in hospitals.[8] In this way, a deaconess's outward appearance was as important to a public acceptance of her as a trained nurse as were her actions. Furthermore, according to historian Anna Sticker, the distinct, modest, but dignified outward appearance of a uniformed nurse reinforced an acknowledgment of her professional role as nurse and deaconess.[9]

Need for Specificity

A specific uniform policy to clearly identify each practitioner as a qualified trained nurse and member of the newly created Protestant nursing order was necessary for the placement of nurses in hospital and community nursing. Dark blue was chosen by the Protestant order as the predominant color. In contrast, Catholicism was strongly associated with "popish" black. For this reason, there was reluctance to accept black for the overcoat, hat, and umbrella.[10] As a member of the Protestant nursing order, the dress needed to show the deaconess's purpose, which was Christian service to the poor in the spirit of Evangelical love. Therefore, the uniform had to look modest and serviceable. It had to be rugged enough (and washable) to wear well despite the hard work required of a nurse, but without resembling the attire of a menial servant woman. Conversely, the uniform could not make the wearer look too refined, suggestive of a higher social class, because then it would appear to be unsuitable for the nature of the nurses' work.[11]

Contemporary Mores

The complex uniform requirements were necessary because early nineteenth-century society was still rigidly divided into social classes. Upward mobility, as is known today, did not exist. A person was born to his social place, was raised to conform to his class expectations, and accepted his station in life. Historically, up to the turn of the eighteenth century, some statutes prohibiting behavior indicative of upward social class movement had been in effect. For example, in some areas dress laws reserved to aristocrats only the right to wear velvet and silk. Also, members of the lower class were prohibited from wearing hats. Their headgear was limited to a cap for men and cap or scarf for women. Villagers could not dress as townspeople; instead, they wore work clothes during the week and on Sunday dressed up in their regional costumes.[12]

In the towns and cities, merchants or tradesmen were readily distinguishable by their attire. So were members of other classes and even, to some extent, occupations. For example, among the trades, some ship carpenters still wore heavy, wide-weave, bell-bottom corduroy pants until 1950. In earlier times, dress served to identify the occupation of the wearer and even his rank within the group. For example, the academic gown, at one time worn daily, marked the magister from the baccalaureate. Similarly, the long coat worn by physicians denoted higher status than that indicated by the short coats of surgeons and practical doctors.[13] A cook or maid wore an apron and a head cap, never a hat. Only women from the middle class and above wore hats.[14]

Some dress customs were specific to women because in a male dominated society, tradition demanded easy recognition of a woman's marital status. This distinction by dress was most pronounced among middle and upper classes. In the nineteenth century, outward appearance still differentiated married from unmarried women.[15] Married women were accorded a respect not extended to single women of marriageable age. While a married woman could move about unescorted, public appearance by single women of marriageable age was proper only when they were accompanied by a married woman or an elderly female. Women's place was within the family. Unmarried females occupied themselves appropriately with acceptable designated female work activities, among which were nursing sick household members within the parameters of an extended family.[16]

Family systems were patriarchal. By custom and civil law, the senior male, usually the father, was responsible for all female household members. In turn he was the provider, whom society judged by the extent to which he provided for his family (usually measured by creature comforts, clothing, luxuries, etc.) and by the degree of control, including protection, exercised over the household. Female household members were themselves as much external displays of family values as was their attire and activity. For example, if an unmarried woman, assuming this possibility, were to be gainfully employed outside the home, the patriarch would have been perceived as being (1) no longer in control, (2) unable to provide for his family, and (3) irresponsible, for allowing her to expose herself to the dangers of the world; he would have defaulted on his obligation to protect her.[17]

In this arrangement, women, especially young unmarried females, were indulged in at the price of personal independence. Their clothing was fashionable, colorful, and, depending on family means, expensive. Their dress displayed family wealth, representing the patriarch's economic achievements. Women also dressed to attract attention because their sole objective was to find a suitable mate. To pursue this goal, however, women required protection; thus, they were escorted in public. The availability of family members for this function and the clothing worn by unmarried women, in turn, indicated affordable leisure, a luxury not possible for the lower classes. Working-class people worked to survive. Assuming they were able to afford silk, and such, the working class had no means or help for its upkeep. Females could not be spared to escort the others. Every able body had to work. Their hands were to do work while those of the higher class were protected with gloves. In this culture, obstacles to establishing nursing as an occupation for middle-class, unmarried women were formidable.[18]

Middle-class married women, whose attire (style, brighter colors, more adornments on dress and hat) distinguished them from those unmarried, were afforded greater latitude in personal movement and interaction. Because they were recognizable as being married, they received the respect due their married state. They belonged to their husband and, therefore, even unescorted were not in danger of being molested. They always enjoyed much greater personal freedom than younger single women or older spinsters.[19] Of course, employment for single women was unthinkable.

The external attire and dress etiquette of unmarried females made them unlikely candidates for pioneering employment of women in a respected occupation. Because of these social restrictions, a new standard of dress was needed. An easily recognizable uniform dress that conveyed the proper status and respect for members of the new nursing order became an essential necessity. The nurse's attire had to identify her special role and give her protection when going about her business as a nurse in the public domain.[20] The deaconess-nurse dress, thus, would pave the way for the new profession of nursing.

Design Strategy

A new image of nurses had to be established. According to Sticker, Fliedner solved the problem by "choosing the contemporary dress of a married woman (middle-class townswoman) from the lower Rhineland."[21] This ingenious design greatly changed prevailing pejorative attitudes against respectable women assuming the nurse role. Recognizable by their uniform attire, deaconess nurses successfully withstood public scrutiny, even though their work involved menial labor and put them in close personal contact with male patients, a major taboo at the time. (It was unthinkable to imagine proper women publicly engaged in activity requiring close proximity to the naked body parts of men.)[22] Dressed in uniform, however, Kaiserswerth nurses were accorded the respect they needed to function with a degree of independence as yet unknown by single women.

Fliedner, recognizing the importance of public print to image building, reprinted a previously published article taken from a weekly paper in his *Der Armen und Krankenfreund*. The article praised the deaconess-nurses' appearance as indicative of their competence. To this Fliedner added: "It is overall useful to make known the viewpoints of unbiased

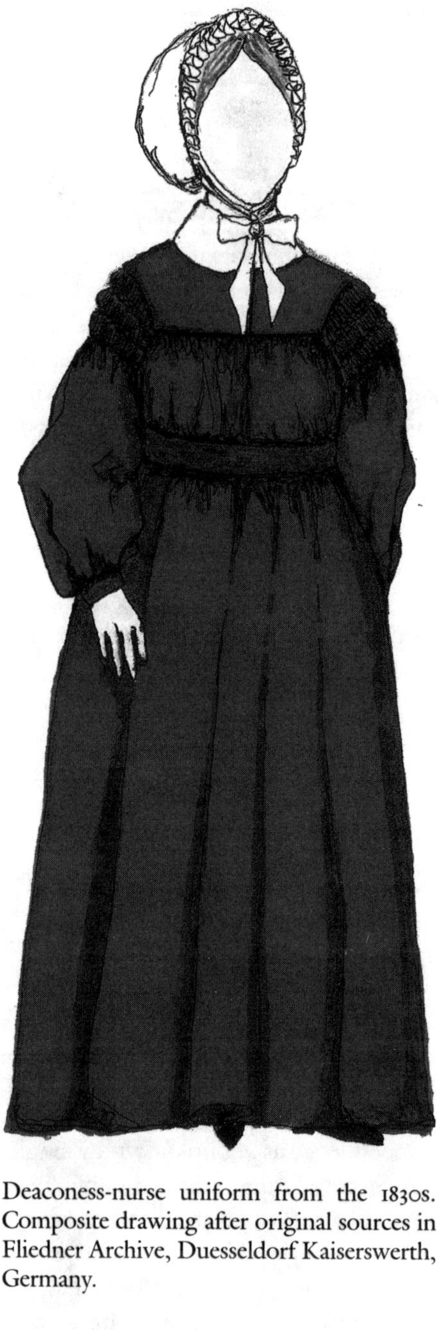

Deaconess-nurse uniform from the 1830s. Composite drawing after original sources in Fliedner Archive, Duesseldorf Kaiserswerth, Germany.

observers, who, as the author, admit to have been prejudiced against the deaconesses, but through observation changed their opinion."[23]

Uniform Description

The uniform of a graduate nurse-deaconess consisted of a blue cotton dress that reached to the feet, blue cotton apron, white snug-fitting cap tied under the chin, white collar, and scarf. The dress was unadorned. The Sunday dress was of the same design and color but made from fine wool cloth. The Sunday cap was made of white net cloth, which was edged by a ruffle of the same cloth for graduate nurses. Stockings were knitted cotton or wool. A black, loose-fitting (to deemphasize body contours) coat completed the outfit. Velvet or fur trim was prohibited. The style had to conform to the designs of the coats made at the Institute.[24]

The Hat

In public, the deaconess wore an accentuated, large-brimmed, black bonnet on top of her cap. The bonnet reflected early-nineteenth-century fashion. Fliedner writes, "The hats are of black silk, follow the design of those made here, are without any adornment, large and fitting enough to protect from the sun and intrusive stares."[25] The hat was most important to preserving the dignity of these young women and conferring ladylike respect upon them. Thus the whole attire, and especially the hat, served to overcome the social class problems. The bonnet's large brim served to protect the nurses not only from general public scrutinizing, but also from intrusive gazing by men, thus forestalling easy encounters that "could lead to temptations for the young women and give rise to scandalous gossip."[26]

Sticker writes that,

> In public appearances, attired with the hat, the deaconess resembled a solid middle class matron. Gertrud Reichardt, the daughter of a physician and the first deaconess nurse, being middle class was used to wearing a hat. Others, however, who came from the lower classes, in conformity with the strict class system, were unaccustomed to wearing a hat.[27]

The addition of a hat in the uniform of a refined, trained nurse afforded her a certain respectability, but did not serve to encourage social climbing. "In view of the quantity, quality, and color of the material used for the whole outfit," Sticker judges the attire to have given deaconesses "a well-

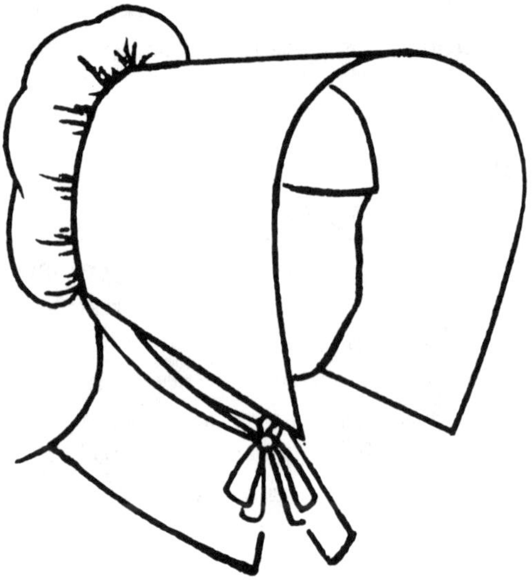

Deaconess-nurse outdoor hat from the 1830s.
Free drawing from textual descriptions.

dressed, conservative middle class appearance that was far above the Prussian norm."[28] Sticker concludes that,

> The hat worn in public . . . conveyed the lady image. . . . Without changing the social order, a revolutionary step had been made. This uniform enabled the unmarried woman, as long as she had committed herself to a five-year service contract with the Deaconess Association, to function unmolested in public pursuit of her nursing occupation.[29]

Policy Compliance

An open letter from Fliedner and his wife Caroline, dated October 1848, demonstrated the importance attributed to compliance with the uniform regulations to all Kaiserswerth deaconesses engaged in distant nursing assignments away from the mother house.[30] Because of noncompliance by some with uniform regulations, the letter admonished the nurses to strictly adhere to the clothing regulations. It continued by reminding them of their promise to obey. The letter unequivocally states:

> Obedience in this case means obeying the uniform regulations. . . . Those of you who are guilty of infractions against the dress regulation will discover that either ignorance of the same, vanity, complacency, carelessness or an inappropriate thriftiness have led you to this action, and you must admit that it can only be helpful to your occupation when you avoid or overcome such errors. The Sunday and everyday dresses, aprons and caps must be of the same color, material, and cut as those you received upon assuming your duties.[31]

The letter further reiterates the need to wear the white collar. For those who owned a black dress, the prohibition to wear it except for special church services or "as a sign of mourning was reinforced."[32] Hat replacements were to be ordered from the mother house.

> Other than this silk hat, and a silk umbrella, perhaps also a simple pouch of black silk, deaconesses are not allowed to wear silk, whether on dresses, aprons, full or half scarves . . . those who especially need to wear a scarf around the neck must wear one made of white linen or cotton. During occasions of extended appearance in public, and also the shortest public appearance in a larger city, the deaconess wears hat and scarf.[33]

The conclusion reminds the deaconesses of their duty to obey the uniform regulation and their commitment to the mother-house policy.

> A dress regulation which gives direction in every way is now even more necessary. . . . We have come to recognize that the present rules, as given in the Hausordnung, while not needing to be changed, nevertheless require more specific instructions and limitations, and expect from all of you in accordance with your promise, compliance and willing obedience with the Institute's specified clothing policy.
>
> Fliedner, Pfr. (Pastor)
> Caroline Fliedner[34]

The Fliedners reacted so vehemently because some deaconesses had made personal changes in their attire and apparently had also voiced dissatisfaction with the strict rules.[35] Sticker writes that two nurses questioned the need for wearing the white collar while attending to all the heavy hospital work, especially early in the morning. In addition to bedside nursing, early morning activities included scrubbing laundry, cleaning vegetables, and stoking stoves. Earlier, Friedericke Fliedner had debated substituting a black scarf instead of the white collar for probationers—at least until they had acquired the habit of keeping themselves clean.[36] These and other notations by Friedericke and Theodor attest to the difficulties encountered in teaching the young women, who usually were of lower-class origins, the paramount importance of the proper wear and care of their prescribed uniform for maintaining the proper public image and, thus, the continued success of the nursing venture.

Sticker writes that requiring full dress upon rising opposed the customary practice, for women in general, of doing morning household chores in a housecoat. "Only later in the morning did she dress fully."[37] But Kaiserswerth nurses had to be fully dressed for public view from early morning to bedtime. The dignified image had to be constantly maintained, even early in the morning when nurses engaged in coarse, dirty household tasks. After all, nurses were always in public view of patients. Exceptions were not and could not be tolerated. Creation of the nurse image was as important, perhaps even more so, than any other factor that created the new nurse.

Probationers

Although probationers could "wear their own clothing during the six months probationary period, unless it is found necessary to acquire a housedress for them," a visitor to Kaiserswerth noticed their distinct appearance.[38] Fredricka Bremer, a Swedish novelist and early feminist, was attracted by the Institute's reputation for training women to assume an occupation and visited Kaiserswerth in 1846. She wrote: "All sisters wear the same clothing consisting of a dark blue cotton thing [dress], a plain white collar, and a simple, white cap. A small white lace on the cap differentiates those not yet invested from those invested, the actual deaconesses."[39]

References in other documents to the white collar, cap, and dark color of the probationers' outer dress show that they were expected to conform only with the general uniform requirements. They could wear their own clothing if it was of dark color and simple style. Most likely their dress did not have to rigidly conform because they worked in the Institute's hospital, were not exposed to the general public, and were not yet permanent members. For them, learning neatness, cleanliness, and simplicity in clothing was more important as a component of their probationary training. As prospective members of an honored group, they also had to learn to take pride in their outward appearance; yet, they were to remain humble, seemingly unaware of dress customs, fashion, and other forms of vanity—indeed, a seemingly paradoxical goal.

Implicit Meaning

On the back of an envelope, Fliedner noted his thoughts on the uniform, its purpose, and its symbolic meaning. The everyday work dress was to distinguish the nurse as representative of the important office of nursing and of the competence required of a professionally trained nurse.[40] Her skills and demeanor set her apart from housemaids, untrained nurse attendants, and idle, middle-class women; her attire symbolized her professional characteristics. Also, the uniform helped the nurse gain entry into households and confer the privileges of a reputable woman, and it exempted her from fashion requirements.[41]

The Sunday dress of the nurse was to be like the work dress because, Fliedner wrote, "she often has to attend to the sick [on Sundays]." Therefore it had to be practical, but also "convey the proper respect in interactions with patients." To honor Sunday and special holidays, however, the dress material was of a better cloth. Fliedner specified a dark blue color because often "patients fear black . . . and because it is extremely gloomy . . . [whereas] dark blue is modest and yet cheerful."[42]

Complete Wardrobe

A one-page document lists the complete wardrobe requirements for a traveling nurse:

Clothing articles, etc., which the traveling sister *takes along*

6 shirts	5 pair shoes and houseshoes
4 slips	1 pair overshoes
2 corsets	4 leg dressings [possibly wet-weather coverings]
3 pair whites [underwear]	2 underjackets
4 pair colored [undergarments]	1 sewing box
4 pair woolen stockings	combs, toothbrush
4 proper dresses	clothing brush
1 sleeping coat	2 black scarves
6 aprons	2 hats
2 black aprons	1 coat
12 scarves	1 umbrella
12 handkerchiefs	1 hat box
6–12 collars	1 suitcase

6–8 caps
3 night jackets
6–12 night caps
1 Bible and 10–12 books
1 other picture
1 travel sack
1 travel satchel
1 notebook or briefcase
1 money pouch
deaconess certificate[43]

It was a substantial wardrobe, befitting a middle-class woman, providing for adequate changes between washings. It allowed the nurse to maintain cleanliness without compromising her busy schedule.

Image Validated

The goal of creating the image of a neat, clean, competent nurse and respectable woman was achieved, as is corroborated by a contemporary writer's description, dated 1850, of a practicing community of nurses in a small town.

> Several days after my request two "sisters," as they are usually called, arrived to give help to the overburdened families. And if already, upon meeting them, my prejudices disappeared, then this occurred even more so upon observing them among the sick. Their hands, their clothing which is most suited for the work, which consisted of a blue dress, white collar and white, simple cap (in winter they wear a black coat), already gave me the certainty that they knew how to do an honest piece of work. Of course, their collar and cap were always gleamingly white, because cleanliness, neatness, and tidiness are their attributes, in hospitals as well as in their personal surroundings.[44]

The dress of a Kaiserswerth deaconess announced her dedication, professionalism, and honorability to the public; as contemporary accounts show, her subsequent behavior and nursing skill confirmed the good reputation her clothing indicated.

Catalyst for Change

Because of Fliedner's brilliant plan to make the attire worn by Kaiserswerth nurses central to the strategy for reforming nursing and women's public role, the nurse uniform acquired singular importance. It became an instrument for change. The uniform established an image of respectability and competence for nurses: a necessary antecedent to societal changes that allowed respectable women to be employed as nurses in public hospitals. The nurse uniform was neither a romantic idea nor mere functional attire, but a powerful catalyst for gaining the acceptance of modern nursing as a reputable occupation and for quietly revolutionizing women's status in early-nineteenth-century Prussia. In turn, the image of nursing established by Kaiserswerth deaconesses in Germany laid the foundation for Nightingale's advancement of nursing in the 1860s.

IRENE SCHUESSLER POPLIN, PHD, RN, CS
Associate Professor
Division of Nursing
Midwestern State University
3410 Taft Blvd.
Wichita Falls, Tex. 76308-2099
Phone: (817) 689-4600

Notes

1. For a more complete history of the origins of modern nursing at Kaiserswerth, see Irene Schuessler Poplin, "A Study of the Kaiserswerth Deaconess Institute's Nurse Training School in 1850–1851: Purposes and Curriculum" (PhD diss., University of Texas at Austin, 1988). German primary and secondary sources used in this analysis were translated by I. Poplin into English. Many primary documents handwritten in German script required additional transliteration. All primary documents are housed at the Fliedner Archive, Diakonissenanstalt, Kaiserswerth, Germany (hereafter F. A.).

2. Extensive contextual reading on nineteenth-century German nursing and the status of women is found in Anna Sticker, *Die Entstehung der neuzeitlichen Krankenpflege* [*The Origin of Modern Nursing*] (Stuttgart: W. Kohlhammer, 1960) (hereafter *Krankenpflege*); Martin Gerhardt, *Theodor Fliedner,* 2 Vols. (Duesseldorf-Kaiserswerth: Diakonissenanstalt, 1937). Susan Reverby, *Ordered to Care: The Dilemma of American Nursing, 1850–1945* (Cambridge, Mass.: Cambridge University Press, 1987) extensively examines the unique dilemma of women's private and public role and the aspirations for nursing as a female profession in the United States.

3. Reverby, 49.

4. Theodor Fliedner, *Erster bis Sechzehnter Jahresbericht* [First to Sixteenth Annual Report] 1 Januar 1836–1 Januar 1853, Jahresberichte File, F. A.

5. Ibid.; Florence Nightingale, in an anonymous monograph (her first publication) on Kaiserswerth written on Fliedner's request in 1850 after her first visit to the Institute, expounds in some detail on the idea. [Nightingale], *The Institution of Kaiserswerth on the Rhine* (1851; reprint, Duesseldorf-Kaiserswerth: Diakonissenanstalt, 2nd ed., 1959), 1–32.

6. "Deaconess" and "nurse," as used by Fliedner in relation to dress, are synonyms.

7. Theodor and Caroline Fliedner to Deaconesses, "Kleiderordnung fuer die Diakonissen der Anstalt zu Kaiserswerth, fuer Helene Schirp" [Dress policy for the deaconesses of the Kaiserswerth Institute], Oktober 1848, Kleiderordnung File, F. A. This is a letter addressing all deaconesses. The title [Clothing Policy for H. Sch.], however, on a separate paper, is not a letter of salutation but a clothing policy for the named deaconess. It seems that Fliedner, at times, used a single document for multiple purposes.

8. Both functioned as Lady Superintendents of the order and Institute. They were also matron and clinical director of the hospital and nursing school. Undated handwritten note from Theodor Fliedner on used flattened envelope addressed to "Pastor Fliedner . . . at Kaiserswerth." (Postage stamp on envelope reads "8.3" for day and month.) Caroline Fliedner signed her first name with the letter *C.* Her husband spelled it with the letter *K.* Documents show either of the two spellings. Text in this article follows Caroline's usage; references cite the name as used in the specific document. Note that the Fliedner Archive holds a Karoline Fliedner file named K. F.

9. Anna Sticker, ed., *Friedericke Fliedner,* 2nd ed. (Neukirchen: Neukirchener Verlag des Erziehungsvereins, 1961), 168, 171.

10. Undated handwritten note from Theodor Fliedner, "Bedeutung der dunkelblauen Farbe" [Meaning of the dark blue color], Kleiderordnung File, F.A.

11. Undated handwritten note to Kleiderordnung from Theodor Fliedner, Kleiderordnung File, F.A.

12. A. R. L. Gurland, "Wirtschaft und Gesellschaft im Uebergang zum Zeitalter der Industrie," in *Propylaen Weltgeschnichte,* ed. Golo Mann (Berlin: Propylean, 1960), 282.

13. Gurland, 280–85; see also Heinrich Kullmauer and Albert Meher, "Short Robed Surgeon Catherizes a Patient," illustration from *Sketchbook,* courtesy of the Trustees of the British Museum in Ann Carmichael and Richard Ratzau, *Medicine: A Treasury of Art and Literature* (New York: Hugh Lauter Levin Assoc., Inc., Macmillan, 1991), colorplate 39, 119.

14. *Der Brockhaus in Zwei Baenden* (Wiesbaden: F. A. Brockhaus, 1977), 364.

15. Sticker, *Friedericke,* 168.

16. Ibid.

17. *Brockhaus,* 364.

18. Helmut Bleiber and Guenter Hildebrandt, *Bourgeoisie und Buergerliche Umwaelzung in Deutschland, 1789–1871* (Berlin: Akademic, 1977), 48–50.

19. Sticker, *Krankenpflege,* 35; Gerhardt, 2:550–51.

20. Undated handwritten draft of "Kleiderordnung" by Theodor Fliedner, Kleiderordnung File, F. A.

21. Sticker, *Friedericke,* 171.

22. Theodor Fliedner, *Hausordnung der Diakonissenanstalt* [Houserules for the Institute], 1837, Fliedner File, F. A. Theodor Fliedner's file omits Theodor. Signed letter from Friedericke Fliedner to Theodor Fliedner, 14 June 1839, Friedericke Fliedner, Briefe [letters] File, F. A.

23. "Der fuenfwoechentliche Aufenthalt zweier Diakonissen aus Kaiserswerth in Borgholzhausen" [The Five Week Stay of Two Deaconesses from Kaiserswerth in Borgholzhausen] (1850; reprint *Der Armen und Krankenfreund,* Maerz 1850): 1–4.

24. Theodor Fliedner, "Kleiderordnung," Kleiderordnung File, F. A.; Sticker, *Friedericke,* 170; Theodor Fliedner, "Notizbuch" [Notebook], F. A.

25. Theodor Fliedner, "Kleiderordnung," Kleiderordnung File, F. A.

26. Ibid.; handwritten remarks by Friedericke Fliedner on "Kleiderordnung," Kleiderordnung File, F. A.

27. Sticker, *Friedericke,* 171. For Reichardt, the uniform lowered her social-class standing. Most of the others, who came from a lower social class, gained a higher status.

28. Ibid.

29. Ibid.

30. Theodor Fliedner and Caroline Fliedner, "Kleiderordnung," Kleiderordnung File, F. A.

31. Ibid.

32. Ibid.

33. Ibid.

34. Ibid.

35. "Pflegerinnenbuch" [*Nurses Registery Book*], F. A.; Sticker, *Friedericke,* 158.

36. Friedericke Fliedner, "Bemerkungen" [Remarks], Friedericke Fliedner File, F. A.; Theodor Fliedner, "Kleiderordnung," Kleiderordnung File, F. A.

37. Sticker, *Friedericke,* 172.

38. Theodor Fliedner, "Tagesordnung" [Daily Schedule], Tagesordnung File, F. A.

39. Fredricka Bremer, "Kaiserswerth am Rhein 1846," reprinted in Sticker, *Krankenpflege,* 341–46.

40. Theodor Fliedner, "Kleiderordnung," Kleiderordnung File, F. A.

41. Handwritten remarks by Theodor Fliedner, "Kleiderordnung," Kleiderordnung File, F. A.; Johann Christian Friederich Burk, ed., *Der Christenbote* 28, no. 9 (14 July 1839): 280; letter from Marie Schaefer, Kaiserswerth, to Burk in Grossbotwar, 11 June 1839, Briefe File, F. A.; letters from Theodor Fliedner, Kaiserswerth, to Burk, Fliedner File, F.A.

42. Handwritten note by Theodor Fliedner, on "Kleidung" [Clothing], Kleiderordnung File, F. A.

43. Undated handwritten list, "Kleiderstuecke etc., welche die reisenden Schwestern mitnehmen" [Clothing Items to be Taken along by Traveling Sisters], Kleiderordnung File, F. A.

44. "Der fuenfwoechentliche," 1–4.

INTERNATIONAL NURSING HISTORY CORRESPONDENCE

Nursing and Medical Care in Finland from the Eighteenth to the Late Nineteenth Century

The Background for the Introduction of Nurses' Training in Finland in 1889, with Some Comparisons with Developments in Sweden

MARIANNE TALLBERG
Tampre University

Early in the eighteenth century many of the existing *hôpitaux* in France were reorganized so as to cater exclusively for patients regarded as curable. In Germany new hospitals were built for this purpose. These developments were not solely a consequence of a change in the ideological climate; they proved to be a precondition for progress in medicine and surgery and for training physicians in the new methods of treatment.[1] The influence of such thinking on the continent led to the establishment of a new hospital system in Sweden.

This article is a slightly modified version of the original printed in the *Scandinavian Journal of History* 14 (1989) under the same title. We are grateful to Marianne Tallberg and the *Scandinavian Journal of History* for their permission to reprint.

Nursing History Review 2 (1994): 169–190.

The First New Hospitals

The first new hospital in Sweden, the Royal Seraphim Hospital in Stockholm, opened in 1752. Because of economic difficulties it initially only had eight beds, but the numbers increased rapidly, and had reached thirty-six by 1755. The hospital was financed by various taxes and collections from the whole kingdom, but neither the population nor the authorities in Finland were happy about collecting donations for a hospital in Stockholm, even if sick people from the whole country had the right to seek admission to it.[2] The joint effort of the Åbo region succeeded in convincing parliament that a hospital should be established at Åbo, partly in the interests of the sick and partly in order to meet the need for training physicians.[3]

The county hospital at Åbo was opened in March 1759. The Finns were thus able to obtain a hospital of their own almost ten years before it was permitted to establish county hospitals in the rest of the kingdom.[4] A further six county hospitals were opened in Finland before this part of the old Swedish kingdom was incorporated into the Russian empire in 1809.[5] These hospitals were initially supervised by two knights of the Order of the Seraphim, and the administration was enlarged in 1776 by the addition of a director-general of all hospitals in the kingdom.[6]

The Division of Labor within Finnish Hospitals

The earliest hospitals functioned for many years without regulations or instructions. A doctor of medicine, a barber-surgeon, and an administrator were generally employed at each hospital, and in the early years the hospital doctor was often also the provincial physician.[7] A short time after Finland's incorporation into the Russian empire, the hospital doctors undertook to look after the hospitals alone, with only occasional assistance from a barber-surgeon if they were not qualified surgeons themselves, in return for receiving both salaries. This measure placed an overwhelming burden of work on the shoulders of the hospital doctors with the expansion of the hospital system later in the nineteenth century.[8]

The hospitals were run by a management board, of which the county governor was an *ex officio* member.[9] Ultimate responsibility for admitting a patient rested with this board after the hospital doctor had advised whether the illness was curable or not. The instructions issued for all hospitals in the kingdom in 1794 defined the duties of the hospital doctors to include, in addition to their purely medical tasks, ensuring that the administrator kept the hospital clean and aired and that the food and drink produced for the patients were of good condition and well prepared.[10] The administrator was responsible for the hospital's finances and provisions and for the upkeep of its buildings. He also engaged and supervised the workman, the wardress, and the maid in accordance with the terms of the servants' statute. The wardress was in a special position in that she could not be engaged or dismissed without the consent of the hospital doctor, but at the same time she was, as a servant, subordinate to the administrator.[11] The hospitals were subject to a system of dual supervision: The hospital doctor checked that the administrator was performing his duties properly, but the administrator was also instructed to check that patients were visited daily by the doctor and that they received diligent and appropriate care from the wardress.[12]

These regulations were never officially revoked, but they were gradually changed as new regulations were added from the late 1850s.[13] The hospitals may be regarded as under the leadership of the doctors from the 1850s onward.[14]

Descriptions of female personnel given in hospital budgets and regulations varied considerably. The regulations of 1796 for Åbo County Hospital refer to wardresses,[15] while the 1802 budget of Tavastehus Hospital talks about employing maids *or* nurses.[16] It was only toward the end of the nineteenth century that the word *maid* gradually came to mean washerwoman/charwoman,[17] while the term *wardress* increasingly gave way to *nurse* when describing the personnel which cared for the patients.[18] The male employees who looked after male patients who were mentally ill or suffering from venereal disease were initially called *workmen* or *warders*,[19] but were later described as *male nurses*.[20] Hospitals also eventually came to employ lodgekeepers and porters.[21] At the New Surgical Hospital in Helsinki, it was the porters who assisted the doctors in the outpatient clinic.[22]

The Duties of Wardresses at the End of the Eighteenth Century

The regulations of Åbo County Hospital, one of the first to be issued in 1796, described both the duties and the rights of wardresses. This shows that the tasks performed by the wardresses were beginning to be regarded as more important than the work carried out by the other servants.

With regard to the care and nursing of the sick, the wardress was subordinate to the hospital doctor and was to follow his instructions carefully and to give the patients all the assistance they required. This included distributing prescribed medicines and ensuring that the patients took them, but she was not allowed to administer any medicine on her own initiative.

Under the supervision of the administrator, the wardress was to take charge of the patients' own clothes and ensure that they had been washed when the patients were discharged from the hospital. Her duties included lighting the fires in the hospital, airing its rooms, sweeping its floors, smoking its rooms with juniper or vinegar, attending to the washing of the patients' eating utensils and laundry, and generally ensuring that the hospital was tidy and clean.[23]

If these regulations are compared with those issued for the Royal Seraphim Hospital in 1788, striking differences become apparent.[24] The whole running of the Royal Seraphim Hospital, except for the actual medical care, was contracted out. The private contractor also employed the "subordinate personnel," a group which included the wardresses. This is probably the reason why the stipulations relating to wardresses were more detailed in the 1788 regulations for the Royal Seraphim Hospital. She was to care for patients "gently, tenderly and diligently," she was not to leave her ward in daytime, and she was to come immediately at nighttime if one of the patients rang for her. She was not to force any patient to assist her, but if any did so voluntarily, this was permitted. She was solely responsible for cleaning the hospital, lightning its fires, and airing its rooms, but she could ask the workmen to help her with bathing the patients. The workmen also assisted in dressing external injuries and at operations.

The Development of Health Care under the Collegium Medicum

A royal charter of 1663 had conferred on the Collegium Medicorum, a body founded at the initiative of a group of physicians in Stockholm, the responsibility for supervising the practitioners of all forms of medical care in the kingdom.[25] In this connection, the charter explicitly mentioned surgeons, apothecaries, and midwives, but not nurses, who did not exist in Sweden at that time. With the creation of the Health Commission in 1737, the college came for a time to be uninvolved in many of the important events that occurred in the development of medical care, including the introduction of the hospital system, whose management was later taken over by the Order of the Seraphim guild.[26]

The incorporation of Finland within the Russian empire in 1809 created new economic and administrative problems for the country's health care. The county hospitals, except for that in Åbo, had partly been financed by the Order of the Seraphim guild, and provincial physicians had also received their remuneration from Sweden. Physicians, surgeons, and midwives had completed their training in Stockholm, because some kinds of medical institutions—for example, maternity hospitals—did not exist in Finland. Moreover, the country was ravaged by syphilis, and the medical care of both the mentally ill and prisoners had been neglected.[27]

During the first years after 1809, health questions were dealt with by the chancery of the Economics Department.[28] In 1811 the Imperial Medical College was founded, and it assumed the tasks previously carried out by the Swedish *Collegium Medicum* and the Order of the Seraphim guild.[29]

The number of hospitals in Finland increased greatly during the first half of the nineteenth century, but the population also doubled during this period. However, from 1850 until the middle of the 1880s, the number of patients treated in hospital each year did not grow, except during the famine years of the late 1860s. The proportion of syphilitic patients was high; at some times they occupied half of the beds in the county hospitals alone.[30] Conditions in the hospitals were not particularly pleasant. The affluent usually had no choice in the case of mental illness, but they arranged for private care in the case of somatic illnesses.[31] At a later stage, the general hospitals offered the higher ranks of society private rooms, better food, and better service, in return for higher fees. The patients mainly came from the lower social groups, and the problem for them was that the number of free beds did not always match demand.[32]

The Nurses at Nineteenth-Century Hospitals

It remained the task of the administrator to ensure that the nurse "faithfully, diligently and properly fulfills her duties."[33] A proposed set of regulations for hospitals recommended that nurses be middle-aged, healthy, clean, serious-minded, and kindly persons of well-attested good character.[34] Elias

Lönnrot, the creator of the Finnish national epic *Kalevala,* had a similar view of what was required to make a good nurse, but he added that she should also be sober and that older women should be used in the treatment of epidemic illnesses.[35]

The duties of nurses were not limited to caring for the patients, washing, and cleaning. She was also sometimes involved in collecting, cleaning, and drying medicinal plants,[36] in preparing medicaments, and in distributing medicine to the patients.[37] The head of the Imperial Medical College, Gabriel Bonsdorff, reported after his tour of inspection in 1818 that nurses were not always up to performing their duties. Conditions in old Finland, which had been annexed by Russia in 1743 and only reunited with the rest of Finland in 1812, were quite worrying; Bonsdorff noted, for example, that at Viborg the patients were never washed, not even when they first arrived at the hospital.[38]

Inventories of equipment kept in the rooms of individual hospital employees can give us some insight into the division of labor among the personnel. For example, the doctor had the operating table and the cabinet containing medical instruments in his room, while the workman had an axe, a hammer, and a saw in his. The nurse's room was very well stocked. The presence of portable bathtubs, washing bowls, and foot basins show that she was responsible for the personal hygiene of patients. The shaving bowl with brush and razor indicate that it was she, not the workman, who shaved the male patients. The number of vomit bowls, enema syringes, and bedpans in her room suggest that these items were frequently used. The presence of scissors for cutting linen dressing, drawers for lint and bandages, an instrument with which plaster was applied, a phlebotomy instrument, and syringes for administering injections indicate that she was also involved in more complex medical tasks. The catheters, however, were listed among the doctor's instruments. The nurse's room also contained the dustpan and brush and the censer used for dispersing stale air in the wards.[39]

The regulations for hospitals issued later in the nineteenth century by the Medical Board (formerly Imperial Medical College) only mentioned in passing that nurses should obediently follow the instructions given by the doctor, but principally placed them under the authority of the administrator.[40] It was first in the budget for the New Surgical Hospital in Helsinki that a statement appears to the effect that nurses should preferably have obtained some form of secondary education and should not therefore be "burdened with rough or menial tasks."[41]

The Training of Deaconesses

One of the most wealthy philanthropists of nineteenth-century Finland, Aurora Karamsin, was highly religious and was fascinated by the deaconess idea. She had come into contact with the training of deaconesses at the *Evangelische Hospital* in St. Petersburg, which opened in 1859, and wanted to found a deaconess-house in Finland.[42] Aurora Karamsin was a member of the Women's Association in Helsinki, and in 1861 she proposed that the association should undertake the task of planning, opening, and managing a deaconess-house in Helsinki, which she would finance. Zachris Topelius, a poet and university teacher who was also the association's secretary, discussed this proposal with Uno Cygnaeus, among others. Cygnaeus, the "father" of primary education in Finland, advised against the idea.[43] He had obtained a negative impression of Fliedner's deaconess model during a visit to Germany.[44] Aurora Karamsin's proposal came to nothing, because the degree of support for it within the Women's Association was not sufficiently strong and enthusiastic.[45] At the same time, family concerns took Karamsin to Paris for several years. During her absence, two Finnish women trained as deaconesses in St. Petersburg.

Some years later, the famine of 1867 gave a flying start to the deaconess-house in Helsinki. Aurora Karamsin was to fulfill two goals, one was to meet the need for care for the poor and sick, the other was to provide women, including those from the educated classes, with an opportunity for "self-sacrificing work in the service of humanity."[46] It proved difficult to recruit would-be deaconesses. The few applicants were mainly working-class women or the daughters of peasants. The time was clearly not yet ripe, with a few exceptions, for attracting upper-class women into training as deaconesses.[47] In contrast to the situation in Stockholm, where deaconesses worked at Sabbatsbergs Hospital, the general hospital in Helsinki did not want to employ deaconesses.[48] This reluctance may have been caused in part by the strong home-mission religiosity at the deaconess-house; there was a reluctance to allow religious propaganda at the general hospital.[49]

The Medical Profession's Need for "Auxiliaries"

Since 1841 Finnish doctors had been organized in The Finnish Medical Society (*Finska Läkaresällskapet*), and they kept in touch with each other partly through its meetings and partly through its published proceedings and the Newsletter for Physicians and Pharmacists. From 1866 onward, the society arranged a general conference, at which topical questions were discussed on a biennial basis.[50] At this time, there were no more than 125 physicians in Finland, and it is therefore hardly surprising that Professor Jakob August Estlander suggested that parish clerks might assist the medical profession by disseminating information about how, for example, leg ulcer ought to be treated. The possibility that parish clerks might act as barber-surgeons had been discussed on earlier occasions. It was also proposed at the conference that the assistance of "other suitable persons" should be sought, but no attempt was made to define whom these persons might be. Providing such assistance had formally been one of the tasks of the bath attendants' guild,[51] but there appears to have been no cooperation between them and the physicians.[52]

At the conference in 1869, postponed for a year because of the famine and epidemics, it was noted that the so-called better classes did not use the country's hospitals for either venereal or epidemic diseases. This was regarded as perfectly understandable because, to take one example, the only function of the typhus hospitals had been to hide the most terrible misery from the prosperous members of society.[53] The first occasion on which the doctors really complained about their burden of work and its unfortunate effects on the level of medical care in hospitals was in 1871. The society expressed a desire that there should be an additional physician per county hospital, on the grounds that closer care and attention would speed the recovery of the sick.[54]

It was proposed, in order to prevent trachoma, whose treatment required very individual care, that pastors and primary school teachers become involved in health education.[55] Two years later it was suggested that medical students be sent to "carry out missionary work" in the countryside as "guardians of public health," while midwives should be given a better grounding in childcare.[56] At a later conference, the pastor was again proposed as an auxiliary in the fight against infant mortality.[57]

Konrad Relander, a factory doctor who was himself unable to attend the 1881 conference, sent a letter to the society suggesting that each provincial physician should "aquire an assistant nurse" so that health care might be rationalized. No one present at the conference commented on Relander's proposal, and the resolution adopted by the conference described the shortage of cottage hospitals and "the paucity of doctors" as the main factors inhibiting rational health care in the countryside.[58]

It is clear that doctors could still not think in terms of permanent, trained assistants, even though the first short nursing course for ambulance work was offered to women as early as 1880. It is also surprising that Russia did not exert a greater influence on the development of health care in Finland. In large parts of Russia, the provincial doctors who worked in public health care had the assistance of both male and female barber-surgeons.[59]

The View Taken by Finnish Physicians of the Competence of Women in the Medical Sphere

There are many examples that show that doctors did not value nurses very highly during the nineteenth century. One doctor, when discussing the maintenance of order in his hospital, referred to the presence of "several women and a workman, who themselves need to be supervised."[60] Another comment was that when country doctors sought a nurse for their patients, they usually got "an old woman broken by age" who saw the doctor as a competitor, since she had long been involved in providing quack remedies.[61]

Physicians were aware that midwives did not receive a good training, but midwives were also regarded as not always being as conscientious, reliable, and tenderhearted as they ought to be. Women were also criticized for not always being capable of administrating vaccinations properly.[62] "An end to all controls and the flourishing of quack medicine" was another comment about the situation when women were responsible for providing pharmaceutical supplies.[63]

In 1871 women obtained the right to study medicine at the University of Helsinki, a development that prompted Professor Fredrik Saltzman to observe that the notion that women were suited to be physicians represented an "exaggeration" of female emancipation.[64] He did not begrudge women the possibility of becoming physicians, but believed that it went against their calling in life and that they did not have time during their upbringing to acquire the necessary attributes. He took vaccination as an example that demonstrated that women were unsuited to work in the countryside, that is to say were unable to cope with the difficult conditions involved. In his opinion, the standard had declined since vaccinations had started to be administered by women.[65]

The Need for Educated Nurses Becomes Apparent

The Finnish association for the care of wounded and sick soldiers was founded in 1877, and its first task was to send an ambulance to assist at the front during the Russo-Turkish war. There were no trained nurses in Finland, and the association therefore borrowed two deaconesses from the deaconess-house in Helsinki. The first real nurses in Finland were later trained by Professor J. A. Estlander for the guards battalion's hospitals, which was taken over by the Red Cross that same year.[66]

The experiences gained in connection with sending an ambulance to the front in the Caucasus led the association's annual conference in 1879 to authorize its chairman to negotiate with some of the hospitals in Helsinki about the training of nurses. Applicants who were willing to sign a five-year contract to serve in the event of war received a daily allowance, while others were able to take the course at their own expense.[67] The course, which took place in the department of surgery at the clinical institute, was made up of seven weeks of theoretical study followed by one month of practical work as an assistant nurses in a ward. Similar courses were offered in 1882 and 1884, and at the association's annual meeting in 1885, Professor Saltzman proposed that a further course should be offered since the previous ones had proved useful. The entrance requirements for the courses were that applicants should have completed their primary education, that they should have a reasonably strong constitution, and that they should have reached adulthood. The observation that each applicant's "character" should be investigated shows that it was not envisaged that the applicants would be women from the educated classes.[68]

The Finnish Medical Society Begins to Take an Interest in Nurses' Training

At the Finnish Medical Society's conference in 1883, Konrad Relander proposed that the provincial physicians should be assisted during epidemics by "literate, itinerant male nurses," who had received six to eight weeks' training.[69] This question was now regarded as sufficiently important to justify the appointment of a three-man committee to investigate the proposal.

The committee reported back to the conference two years later. In its report, it observed that Relander had in effect proposed the creation of "a kind of an assistant physician." The committee believed that these itinerant male nurses might easily move from providing "care" to offering "treatment," that is to say to practicing quack medicine. The committee therefore preferred the creation of a small group of "specially trained female nurses," whom the medical board could place wherever they were needed during epidemics. It was agreed during the ensuing discussion that the training of these nurses ought to last three to six months and that the completion of primary education should be a condition for admission. Professor Saltzman supported courses of six months' duration on the grounds that the courses provided by the Red Cross had shown that not even the most gifted students were able to cope with administrating health care on their own after only three months' training.

The doctors attending the conference were now agreed that for a variety of reasons women were better suited to be nurses than men. They were less inclined toward quack medicine because they were more obedient; they provided cheap labor; and it was in accord with "the spirit of the times" to employ women as assistants.[70] A step in the direction of nurses' training had been taken, but the Finnish Medical Society did not put forward its proposal, at least not officially, to the Medical Board.[71]

Women's Position in the Finnish Society

It was the simple, uneducated woman who worked in the hospitals during the nineteenth century. What was the Finnish woman from the educated classes doing in the middle of the century?

She has been the subject of a variety of rather conflicting descriptions. In his book *Herrskapsfolk* [Gentlefolk], K. J. Wirilander describes her as taking no part even in household tasks, which were regarded as unsuitable for fine people.[72] The upper-class women portrayed in the diary kept by the artist Albert Edelfelt's sister during the 1880s are hardly any more industrious. An exception was "poor Sophie," who worked as a clerk.[73] In contrast, the women who lived in the country vicarages were often described as industrious and as possessing nursing skills. Many pastors acquired a medical library, and it was not unusual that their wives looked after one of the more seriously ill parishioners in the vicarage guest room.[74] The Swedish upper-class woman is described in Angela Rundquist's doctoral thesis as an "efficient administrator of the home," and it is quite possible that the same epithet could be applied to some of the women who lived in the manor houses of Finland.[75]

Fredrika Runeberg observes in the memoirs she wrote about her youth that to work for payment was regarded at this time as highly humiliating, indeed as a source of real shame for a girl who wished to number herself among the so-called better class of people. It is noteworthy that Fredrika Runeberg herself, as the wife of Finland's national poet J. L. Runeberg, later had so much housework to do that she seldom had time to write.[76] Another nineteenth-century writer Sara Wacklin, began to support herself at an early age by engaging in one of the few acceptable occupations for an educated woman, namely teaching. She ran a boarding school, the only form of schooling available to many middle- and upper-class girls before girls' schools became widespread.[77]

From the 1840s onward, women in many parts of the country were strongly influenced by the pietism preached by Paavo Ruotsalainen. This movement brought together women from different classes and emancipated them so that they followed the dictates of their own consciences rather than those of their husbands. On the other hand, pietism prevented Finnish women from becoming acquainted with the movement which in other countries was making women aware of the question of their social rights. Moreover, J. V. Snellman's national patriotic movement did not really attract the support of Finnish women until the 1880s.[78]

Several women's associations were founded during the 1840s and 1850s. Some of them, including the association in Borgå established at the initiative of Fredrika Runeberg, supported schools for girls from impoverished families, while others devoted themselves to other forms of activity.[79]

The women's association in Åbo ran a children's home whose goal was to educate "children of the female sex to be competent domestic servants." When the girls reached the age of fifteen they were employed by the members of the association's executive committee to receive their final training.[80] Those who had an aptitude for nursing appear subsequently to have been employed, at the recommendation of the families with whom they had lived, as nurses at the county hospital in Åbo.[81] This was a "feudal" way of involving women from the educated classes in health care.

The Education of Women and the Range of Occupations Open to Them

There was thus a difference, for the woman, between taking paid employment and being involved in philanthropic activities. In 1856 Johan Vilhelm Snellman, the leader of Finland's national revival, wrote in the *Literary Review* that "a man will never, absolutely never, love an independent and self-sufficient woman."[82] This seems to have been a generally accepted view among men, and it is hard to believe that a young girl who still entertained hopes of marriage would have voluntarily sought to pursue a profession.

A woman who did not wish to be employed under the terms of the servants' statute was not faced with a wide choice of occupations.[83] To be a governess or companion were options for educated women who did not want to be dependent on a relative. The first vocational training for women was provided at the teacher-training institute at Jyväskylä, which opened in 1863. It was a socially acceptable vocation, but it did not improve a woman's prospects on the marriage market. The postal service began to employ women in 1864, but the numbers employed in state institutions were still so small in the 1880s that this can hardly be described as a solution to the problem. Local government also provided few openings.[84] There was also a considerable reluctance on the labor market to employ women of high social rank.[85]

Women, both in the Swedish-speaking and the Finnish-speaking camps, who worked for the emancipation of their sex devoted a lot of energy to improving the basic education of girls, since such an improvement was a precondition for active involvement in society. However, it was not until the 1880s that a sustained effort was made to establish a secondary school for Finnish-speaking girls. The initiative was taken by a group of women in Kuopio, led by the author Minna Canth. Much debate and polemics ensued in the press, in which Finnish-speaking women were particularly active. In some contributions to the debate the issue at stake was extended to include the right to an academic education, but the question of vocational training was not discussed.[86] The situation is illuminated by Minna Canth's observation after she had read a Swedish pamphlet called *Quinnofrågan* [Women question]: "I have read with great interest of the efforts made by women in Sweden. How apathetic we Finnish women are compared to them!"[87]

The Educated Woman as a Nurse

Fredrika Bremer's novel *Hertha* prompted considerable debate when it was published in 1856 in Sweden. Many people regarded the book as immoral because its heroine, Hertha, nurses a young man with burns on his knee. Snellman devoted a lot of attention to the book in the *Literary Review* and strongly criticized its feminist tendencies.[88] He probably expressed the common attitude of his age toward nursing when he made the following patronizing observation: "A chap can probably put a plaster on himself in the case of knee injuries of this kind and such help as he might require can be obtained from the first old woman to come along in return for a few coppers." Fredrika Bremer was read everywhere in Finland where Swedish was known, and her opinion was defended by Fredrika Runeberg.[89] Runeberg described a similar case of nursing in her own novel, *Fru Catherina Boije och hennes döttrar,* without provoking debate, presumably because it was regarded as self-evident that the ladies of the manor, like those of the vicarage, would attend to those who required assistance regardless of whether they needed food, comfort, or nursing.[90]

The idea of the educated woman as a secular nurse was discussed in the Swedish journal *Tidskrift för hemmet* [The Journal for the Home] in 1859. In order to stimulate interest in the subject, Florence Nightingale's book *Notes on Nursing* was translated into Swedish and appeared in 1861, only two years after the original.[91] The editors responsible for *Tidskrift för hemmet* were the same women who encouraged the Swedish Red Cross to invest in the training of nurses from the very outset.[92] In 1866, Emily Rappe was sent on a Red Cross scholarship to study at the Nightingale training school in London.[93] After one year of training, Rappe became matron at the department of surgery at the Uppsala Academic Hospital in 1867 and principal of the nurses-training school founded by the Red Cross.[94]

The Beginnings of Nurses' Training

As head of the department of surgery at the general hospital in Helsinki, Professor Fredrik Saltzman was responsible for planning the New Surgical Hospital. Anna Broms, the young director of a children's home who had probably taken one of the Red Cross's courses, was appointed matron, a post hitherto unknown in Finland.[95] The costs of her nurse's training—one year in Stockholm and Edinburgh—were covered by a scholarship from the Senate.[96] At its annual meeting in 1888, the Red Cross decided to finance five scholarships and the remuneration for one doctor to act as a teacher for a nurses' training course the following year.[97] The agreement with the Surgical Hospital appears to have been an oral one. The only official reference to the training of nurses is in the statement outlining the duties of the hospital's assistant physician, which contains the following stipulation: "to teach the theoretical part of such training for nurses as may be arranged." The statement outlining the matron's duties says nothing about trainee nurses except that the matron should "supervise nurses employed at the institution and teach them the practical aspects of nursing."[98]

The only documentary evidence for the introduction of nurses training are the advertisements that appeared on 12 January 1889 in three newspapers—*Uusi Suometar, Helsingfors Dagblad,* and *Nya Pressen*—that stated that "a course for nurses will begin at the Surgical Hospital on 1 February." Not even the hospital's annual report referred to the training of nurses, even though this training provided the hospital with much-needed labor.[99]

Conclusion

A period of administrative, economic, and social reform began in Finland in the 1860s. As for the 1880s, it is possible to speak of a period of significant change in society, and it was perhaps the more free and idealistic current of thought that contributed to the introduction of nurses' training. It also now became quite clear that the hospital nurse herself had not succeeded in developing the nature of her work and her social position: Neither her training nor her social standing had given her any opportunity to do so.

Why had the educated women of Finland failed to take the initiative in the question of nursing? Riitta Jallinoja poses the same question without being able to give an answer when she asks why the first feminist association was not founded until 1884.[100] By this time national consciousness had become well established among Finnish women, and the association strongly supported the initiative efforts that were being made to secure schooling for girls. However, there would still have been time for women to take the initiative over nurses' training. Did they fail to do so because nursing was regarded as such a "working-class" and uncultivated occupation that the educated woman did not even reflect on the matter? Was it in reality the case that the educated Finnish woman was still so tied to the old society based on rank that she did not want to become more deeply involved in the life of society than the demands of philanthropic activity required? Was she perhaps unable to conceive of looking after in concrete, physical terms of someone from a lower social class, namely that section of the population that in practice used the general hospitals?

It is surprising that, at a time when an increasing number of women were remaining unmarried, Finnish women did not see the potential of a caring profession other than that of a doctor.[101] The pressure exerted by educated, unmarried women, which may be part of the explanation for the efforts of Swedish women to secure the introduction of nurses' training, obviously never became sufficiently strong in Finland to persuade women to take the initiative in this question. The idea that women should have a right to an academic education attracted a measure of support, but there was clearly too little social consciousness and united strength among Finnish women to sustain the introduction of a "new" profession. Minna Canth's observation about "how apathetic we Finnish women are" evidently reflected reality.

If we follow the development of medical care in Finland and the discussion within the country's small medical profession, we can observe the gradual emergence of a perceived need for a new division of labor within the health care sector. The guild system had been abolished, and above all the bath attendants but also the barber-surgeons had long before lost their importance in the field of medical care, except inside the armed forces. The country's doctors repeatedly spoke of their growing need for assistance in the fields of both preventive medicine and medical care. Why, then, were no efforts made to train nurses?

The Finnish medical profession had good contacts abroad, especially with Scandinavia, Central Europe, and Britain, though its contacts with Russia were minimal.[102] Some form of nurses' training was introduced at an early stage in many of these countries.

Did Swedish doctors give negative reports to their Finnish colleagues about nurses' training in Sweden? It is certainly the case that the training organized by the Swedish Red Cross encountered some problems and that the training of the Sophia sisters was only begun with some difficulty in 1884.[103]

In the case of male nurses, the medical profession's fear of competition and quack medicine was quite clearly expressed. Why was the assistance of the educated woman not sought at an earlier stage? Did Finnish doctors regard the activities of the deaconess-house in Helsinki in an unfavorable light or wish to protect their own daughters from strenuous work and the risk of infection? The more liberal currents of thought of the time and the realization that the medical knowledge could not be monopolized if the health of the people was to be improved probably contributed to the changed attitude of Finnish doctors to the idea of an educated nurse.

The credit for initiating secular nurses' training in Finland is to be shared by the Red Cross and Professor Fredrik Saltzman. The latter's negative attitude at an earlier stage to female doctors was not relevant in relation to nurses. A nurse "only" needed to have completed elementary education, not to have matriculated, and was to work in a hospital under the leadership of a doctor, not independently in the countryside. The New Surgical Hospital began to be planned in 1878, and Saltzman was appointed to head the department of surgery in 1882. The unsatisfactory conditions in the old clinic may well explain why he did not introduce training at an earlier stage, despite his positive attitude to courses for war ambulance nurses.

In my efforts to study the emergence of the nursing profession in Finland, I have examined a wide variety of sources: the archive of the Medical Board in Finland; some parts of the archives of the Order of the Seraphim guild and the Swedish Medical Board, as well as several other archives; the proceedings and minutes of the Finnish Medical Society; earlier publications concerning health care in Finland, including legislation relating to this matter; nineteenth-century novels; the writings of Finnish feminists; medical and other journals and newspapers. Many questions remain unanswered, because it was often difficult to find information about nursing and the discussion this subject prompted. The work of the nurse attracted so little attention and clearly had such a low value attached to it that no one wrote about it or felt obliged to keep an official record of her activities.

Marianne Tallberg, RN, MA, PhD
Associate Professor
Tampre University
Enåsvägen 10 c
00200 Helsinki
Finland
Phone: +358-0-675887
Fax: +358-0-6821129

Notes

1. Dieter Jetter, *Grundzüge der Krankenhausgeschichte, 1800–1900* (Darmstadt: Wissenschaftliche Buchgeschellschaft, 1977), 1–50.

2. Otto E. A. Hjelt, *Svenska och Finska Medicinalverkets historia, 1663–1812* (Helsingfors: Helsingfors Centraltryckeri, 1893), 3:3–28.

3. Alexander R. Klossner, *Turun lääninsairaalan vaiheita, 1756–1856. Ensimmäiset 100 vuotta* (Turku: Turun yliopiston julkaisuja, 1956), appendix, 1:1–2, 4; Otto E. A. Hjelt, *Medicinska förhållanden i Åbo på 1750-talet,* Lännetär, vol. 7 (Helsingfors, 1882), 114–51.

4. R. G. Modée, *Utdrag utur alle . . . Publique Handlingar, Placater, Förordningar, Resolutioner och Publicationer* (Stockholm: Lorenz L. Grefing, 1774), 8:7052–53.

5. Hjelt, *Svenska och finska,* 3:83–115.

6. Hjelt, *Svenska och finska,* (1891), 1:353–59.

7. Hjelt, *Svenska och finska,* 3:83–115.

8. *Finska Läkaresällskapets allmänna möte 14–15 September 1871,* Finska Läkaresällskapets Handlingar, vol. 13 (Helsingfors, 1871), appendix, 13:22–23.

9. Hjelt, *Svenska och finska,* 3:83–115.

10. Frans. J. Rabbe, *Finlands Medicinal-författningar* (Helsingfors: G. O. Wasenius, 1837), 1:83–85.

11. Richard Wawrinsky, *Sveriges Lasarettsväsen förr och nu. Ett stycke svensk kulturhistoria* (Stockholm: Författarens Förlag, 1906), 558; Modée, (1746), 2:1582–99; *Samling af de i Storfurstendömet Finland gällande och intill år 1855 utkomne Författningar Sednare delen 1800–1854* (Helsingfors: J. C. Frenckell, 1855), 94–112.

12. Rabbe, 1:94–101.

13. Rabbe (1874), 4:173–76, 218–27.

14. Alexander von Collan, *Finlands Medicinalförfattningar* (Helsingfors: Tidnings and Tryckeri Ab, 1894), 6:68–71.

15. "Reglemente för Åbo Läns Lazarett, Skrifvit och stadfäst af Lazaretts Direction den 1 Maji 1796," in Klossner, 1:57–61. Klossner states that the original copy of this document is in the Swedish national archives, but it can not be located.

16. Rabbe, 1:103–5.

17. Rabbe, 4:260–61.

18. Rabbe, 4:189.

19. Rabbe, 1:103–5.

20. Rabbe, (1846), 3:864–68.

21. Rabbe, 4:25; von Collan, 6:70.

22. Ali Krogius, *Kirurgiska sjukhuset i Helsingfors, 1889–1913. Tillika en återblick på kirurgins utveckling under de sista 25 åren,* Kirurgiska sjukhuset årsberättelse 1913 (Helsingfors, 1915), 1–20.

23. Klossner, 1:57–61.

24. R. G. Modée, *Utdrag utur alle . . . Publique Handlingar, Placater, Förordningar, Resolutioner och Publicationer* (Stockholm: Kongl. Tryckeriet, 1829), 15:135–58.

25. Rabbe, 1:5–21.

26. Hjelt, 1:339–59.

27. Niilo Pesonen, *Terveyden puolesta—sairautta vastaan. Terveyden-ja sairaanhoito Suomessa 1800-ja 1900-luvulla* (Porvoo: WSOY, 1980), 3–24.

28. Pesonen, 21–36.

29. Rabbe, (1839), 2:209–12.

30. *Medicinalstyrelsens årsberättelser,* Finska Läkaresällskapets Handlingar, vol. 8–27 (Helsingfors, 1860–1885).

31. "Om de veneriska besigtningarne," *Notisblad för Läkare och Pharmaceuter* 20, no. 5 (1869): 105 (hereafter cited as *NLP*); "Hungersnödens följder i sanitärt afseende, särskilt sednaste tyfusepidemi," *NLP* 20, no. 5 (1869): 102–11.

32. Rabbe, 4:218–27; von Collan, 5:561–62.

33. Rabbe, 1:94–101.

34. Finland, The National Archives, Medicinalstyrelsens Arkiv 1, *Eab 5, Diarie* no. 524 (1829), but is not to be found in the diary.

35. Elias Lönnrot, *Suomalaisen Talonpojan Koti-Lääkäri* (1856; reprint, Tampere: K. R. Wirtasen Kirjapaino, 1981), 16–17.

36. Finland, The National Archives, Medicinalstyrelsens Arkiv 1, *Eab 5, Diarie no.524* (1829).

37. Finland, The County Archives of Vasa, Vasa Länssjukhus, Arkiv, *Ca 1, styrelsens protokoll,* 25 October 1813.

38. Finland, The National Archives, Senatens Arkiv, Ekonomiedepartementet *16/273 BD* (1818).

39. Finland, The National Archives, Medicinalstyrelsen Arkiv 1, *Eab 22* (1844), inventories at Uleåborg and Kuopio county hospitals *Eab 45* (1867); Medicinalstyrelsens Arkiv 2, annual inventory for Kuopio county hospital *Ee 1* (1856).

40. Rabbe, 4:218–27; von Collan, 5:182–95.

41. von Collan, 6:68–71.

42. Erkki Kansanaho, *Kristen tjänst under ett sekel, Diakonissanstalten i Helsingfors, 1867–1967* (Vasa: Förbundet för svenskt församlingsarbete i Finland, 1967), 18–50.

43. Zacharias Topelius correspondence with Uno Cygnaeus during 1861, Helsinki University Library.

44. Finland, The National Archives, Uno Cygnaeus travel diary, 1859.

45. Alexandra Ramsay, "Huvudstadens hjärta. Den tidiga organiserade filantropin i Helsingfors cirka, 1840–1860" (Unpublished postgraduate diss., Helsinki University, Department of History, 1989), 113.

46. Edvin Wirén, *En sådd i tro och kärlek. Diakonissanstalten i Helsingfors, 1867–1942* (Helsingfors: Schildt, 1942), 54–83.

47. Diakonissanstaltens direktionsprotokoll 1868–1899, the Archives of the Deaconesses' Institution in Helsinki.

48. Otto E. A. Hjelt, *Diakonissanstalten i Helsingfors under åren, 1867–1907* (Helsingfors: Kirjapainoyhtiö, 1908), 71.

49. Wirén, 72; Marius W. af Schultén, *"Den medicinska undervisningen i Paris,"* Finska Läkaresällskapets Handlingar, vol. 21 (Helsingfors, 1879), 183.

50. "Om bensår, dessas orsak och behandling," *NLP* 17, no. 5 (1866), 135–88.

51. Rabbe, 1:192–95.

52. Finska Läkaresällskapets Handlingar, vol. 1–31 (1841–1889), *NLP* 1–4, 5–20 (1849–1852, 1854–1869).

53. "Hungersnödens följder i sanitärt afseende, särskilt sednaste tyfusepidemi," *NLP* 20, no. 5 (1869): 102–11.

54. *Finska Läkaresällskapets allmänna möte 14–15 September 1871,* Finska Läkaresällskapets Handlingar, vol. 13 (Helsingfors, 1871), appendix, 9–29.

55. Ibid.

56. *Finska Läkaresällskapets allmänna möte 28–29 May 1873,* Finska Läkaresällskapets Handlingar, vol. 15 (Helsingfors, 1873), appendix, 42–52.

57. *Finska Läkaresällskapets allmänna möte 11–13 September 1879,* Finska Läkaresällskapets Handlingar, vol. 21 (Helsingfors, 1879), appendix, 28–36.

58. *Finska Läkaresällskapets allmänna möte 1–3 September 1881,* Finska Läkaresällskapets Handlingar, vol. 23 (Helsingfors, 1881), appendix, 39–52.

59. "Mischellen," *St. Petersburger Medicinische Wochenschrift* 1, no. 10 (1876): 7; 1, no. 11 (1876): 9; 3, no. 48 (1878): 400.

60. Finland, The National Archives, Medicinalstyrelsens Arkiv 1, *Memorial 4/35 15 January 1827, diary no. 43/1827, Eab 1.*

61. *Finska Läkaresällskapets allmänna möte 11–13 September 1879,* Finska Läkaresällskapets Handlingar, vol. 21 (Helsingfors, 1879), appendix, 38.

62. "Hvad kan i afseende å barnavården i städerne och på landet uträttas," *NLP* 17, appendix (1866): 168–87.

63. *Finska Läkaresällskapets allmänna möte 1–3 September 1881,* Finska Läkaresällskapets Handlingar, vol. 23 (Helsingfors, 1881), appendix, 43.

64. Von Collan, 5:32.

65. *Finska Läkaresällskapets allmänna möte 28–29 May 1873,* Finska Läkaresällskapets Handlingar, vol. 15 (Helsingfors, 1873), appendix, 31–42.

66. Finlands Röda Kors årsberättelse 1877 och styrelse protokoll 15 November 1877, the Archives of the Finnish Red Cross.

67. Finlands Röda Kors årsmötes protokoll 30 December 1879, the Archives of the Finnish Red Cross.

68. Finlands Röda Kors styrelseprotokoll 28 January and 17 March 1880; 5 December 1882; 27 February and appendix, 15 December 1884; 23 November 1885, the Archives of the Finnish Red Cross.

69. *Finska Läkaresällskapets allmänna möte 13–15 September 1883,* Finska Läkaresällskapets Handlingar, vol. 26 (Helsingfors, 1883), appendix, 119–25.

70. *Förhandlingar vid Finska Läkaresällskapets tionde allmänna möte 28–30 September 1885* (Helsingfors: J. C. Frenckell and Son, 1888), 62–82.

71. Finland, The National Archives, Medicinalstyrelsens Arkiv 1. *Diarier för ankomna brev Aa 55 1885 och Aa 56 1886.*

72. Kaarlo J. Wirilander, *Herrskapsfolk. Ståndspersoner i Finland, 1721–1870* (Nordiska Museets Handlingar, vol. 98, Stockholm, 1982), 51.

73. Berta Edelfelt, diary 1886–1888, the Archives of Svenska Litteratursällskapet. "Poor Sophie" was baroness Sophie Mannerheim, who trained as a nurse around the turn of the century and subsequently played an important role in the development of nurses' training while she was matron at the Surgical Hospital in Helsinki from 1904 to 1928.

74. Anna M. Reinilä, "Lääkintätaito ja-toiminta Suomen pappiloissa," *Kotiseutu* no. 4–5 (1972): 211–17.

75. Angela Rundquist, *Blått blod och liljevita händer. En etnologisk studie av aristokratiska kvinnor 1850–1900* (Stockholm, Carlsons, 1989), 64–66.

76. Fredrika Runeberg, *Anteckningar om Runeberg. Min pennas saga,* ed. Karin Allardt-Ekelund, Skrifter utgivna av Svenska Litteratursällskapet i Finland, vol. 310 (Helsingfors, 1946), 209, 216–17.

77. Sara Wacklin, *Hundrade minnen från Österbotten* (Helsingfors: Holger Schildts Förlagsaktiebolag, 1919), 10–26.

78. Alexandra Gripenberg, *Naisasian kehitys eri maissa 4* (Porvoo: WSOY, 1909), 20–23.

79. Johan L. Birck, *Svenska Fruntimmersföreningen i Jakobstad. Hundra år, 1859–1959* (Jakobstad, 1959), 11–15.

80. F. Holmberg, *Ett sekel i barmhärtighetens tjänst. Fruntimmersföreningen i Åbo, 1849–1949* (Åbo, 1949), 30–31.

81. Adele Selander's letter 1902, Olga Lackström's papers in the Archives of SSY-Sjuksköterskeföreningen i Finland.

82. Johan V. Snellman, "Ur Hertha och Hertha eller En Själs Historia," *Litteraturblad för allmän medborgerlig bildning* 10 (1856): 333.

83. Finlands författningssamling no. 2, 1865; no. 1, 1879; no. 45, 1888; Lucinda Hagman, *Om qvinnouppfostran. Iakttagelser och reflektioner* (Borgå: Werner Söderström, 1888), 13–14.

84. *Kalender öfver Kvinnoarbetet i Finland* (Helsingfors: Finsk Kvinnoförening, 1894), 191, 179–86.

85. Hagman, *Om qvinnouppfostran,* 13–14.

86. Sisko Wilkama, *Naissivistyksen periaatteiden kehitys Suomessa, 1840–1880-luvulla,* Historiallisia tutkimuksia, vol. 23 (Helsinki, 1938), 281–315; Minna Canth, "Naiskysymyksiä," *Valvoja* 4 (1884): 169–76, 288–303; 5 (1885), 492–94.

87. Minna Canth, "Brev till Lilli Leinberg 18 November 1880," in *Minna Canthin kirjeet,* ed. Helle Kannila (Helsinki: Suomen Kirjallisuuden Seura, 1973), 41–43.

88. Snellman, 331–37.

89. Gripenberg, 19.

90. Fredrika Runeberg, *Fru Catharina Boije och hennes döttrar* (Helsingfors: Theodor Sederholms Tryckeri, 1858), 48–49.

91. "Qvinnan och sjukvården," *Tidskrift för hemmet, tillegnad den svenska qvinnan* 1 (1859): 100–109; 3 (1861): 3–23; 7 (1865): 209–15; 8 (1866): 229–36.

92. Sten V. Söderberg, *Svenska Röda Korset, 1865–1965-de första 100 åren* (Stockholm: Svensk Litteratur, 1965), 127–44.

93. Sven G. Sjöberg, *Emmy Carolina Rappe i London, 1866–1867,* Sydsvenska Medicinhistoriska Sällskapets Årsskrift, Supplement 10 (Lund, 1988), 12.

94. Elisabet Dillner, *Sjuksköterskeutbildningen inom svenska Röda Korset åren, 1866–1904* (Stockholm: Albert Bonniers Förlag, 1934), 76.

95. *Finska Qvinnor på olika arbetsområden. Biografiskt album* (Helsingfors, 1892), 249–57.

96. Finland, The National Archives, Allmänna Sjukhusets i Helsingfors Arkiv, Brevkoncept 1 April 1887, Anna Broms kontrakt, *Da3 1887–1890.*

97. Finlands Röda Kors årsmötesprotokoll 20 December 1888, the Archives of the Finnish Red Cross.

98. von Collan, 6:68–69.

99. Fredrik Saltzman, G. von Bonsdorff, and A. V. Nordblad, *Kirurgiska sjukhuset i Helsingfors 1889,* Kirurgiska Sjukhuset årsberättelse 1889 (Helsingfors, 1890).

100. Riitta Jallinoja, *Suomalaisen naisasialiikkeen taistelukaudet* (Porvoo: WSOY, 1983), 32–34.

101. Riitta Jallinoja, "Nainen 1800-luvun murroksessa," in *Nainen historiassa*, ed. Auvo Kostiainen, Historian perintö, Turun yliopiston historian laitos, vol. 10 (Turku, 1984), 139–42; Aarno Strömmer, *Väestöllinen muuntuminen Suomessa*, Väestöpoliittisen tutkimuslaitoksen julkaisuja, A:13 (Tornio, 1969), 43–46.

102. Bertil von Bonsdorff, *Läkare och läkekonst i Finland under 300 år, 1640–1940* (Ekenäs: Ekenäs Tryckeri, 1978), 33–34.

103. Eva Bohm, *Okänd, godkänd, legitimerad. Svensk sjuksköterske-förenings första femtio år* (Stockholm: Svensk Sjuksköterskeförenings Förlag, 1972), 26–31.

DOING THE WORK OF HISTORY

Unity Amidst Difference: The ICN Project and Writing International Nursing History

BARBARA L. BRUSH
School of Nursing
University of Pennsylvania

MERYN STUART
School of Nursing
Faculty of Medicine
University of Ottawa

The International Council of Nurses (ICN) is nearing its one-hundredth anniversary. Organized in 1899 through the combined efforts of Ethel Bedford Fenwick, Lavinia Dock, and others, the ICN's purpose was to establish national nursing councils throughout the world and unite nurses through their work.[1] Borrowing rhetoric from the Constitution of the International Council of Women, the ICN more broadly aimed to "advance the good of humanity through greater unity of thought, sympathy and purpose." The ICN has grown from a "club" of British, American, and German nurses at the turn of the century to a multinational organization representing 106 countries and millions of nurses today.[2]

In celebration of the organization's upcoming centennial, the ICN has commissioned a team of historians from Canada, the United States, and Great Britain to write a scholarly history of the ICN and international nursing.[3] The four-year "ICN Centennial History Project" will study the context in which the ICN was created and within which it developed. Ideas

Nursing History Review 2 (1994): 191–203.

of appropriate relations among nurses, negotiation between nursing and other groups, educational goals, ethical and standards debates, issues in the social and economic conditions of nurses, and the role of women were all part of the history of the organization. The influence of organized nursing as countries around the world became industrialized, nationalized, and radically reorganized through war and changing political and economic alignments will also be considered.

Conceptualizing the ICN

This article will focus on two related aspects of the ICN Centennial History Project: First, methodological and theoretical approaches to writing international history and, second, the use of the ideas of "unity" and "difference" as dichotomous concepts that were always in tension throughout ICN's history. Additionally, as an article about history in the making, this writing represents our thinking-to-date about approaches to international nursing historiography.

We will speculate how and why the ICN has survived and maintained its integrity as a unified body amidst the different and rich mixture of its participant countries, focusing on the first three decades of ICN's development.[4] We will also consider the methodological and theoretical problems and dimensions that arise as well as ways to handle these "problems" in our study. Hence, our discussion will integrate conceptual and practical applications of comparative historical research.

Methodology and International History

One of the most important problems that arises in writing international history is the differing national historiographical contexts that one must necessarily manage in a project of this type.[5] Relatively few international or multinational historical studies in nursing or in women's history exist; thus, we are essentially "breaking new ground." Australian historian Judith Allen explains the problem of writing comparative history in this way:

> Comparative historical analysis within the same nation and period can be treated with doubt, while comparison between countries is often treated with palpable suspicion. The grounds are obvious enough and readily borne out by published instances—the dangers are superficiality, over-generalising that

> does violence to diversities, frequent inaccuracies and an over-reliance on secondary sources—hallmarks of the logistical difficulties facing scholars forced to spread efforts too thinly in too many places.[6]

Allen has also pointed out that local, regional, or national studies have been "privileged" over comparative and international frameworks, particularly with regard to the history of feminism. Scholars have seen local studies as richer and more nuanced than broader analyses. To further complicate matters, American and English feminism have been dominant in terms of the sheer volume of published work; the history of Western feminism, therefore, may be mistakenly interpreted as synonymous with American or English feminism. Many historians of American and English feminism, Allen argues, write "as if they assumed their case study was representative." Criticizing this parochial approach, she asserts that the history of Western feminism may not withstand the scrutiny of comparison.[7]

A second methodological (and political) problem arises because the ICN researchers are white, well-educated, English-speaking women attempting to capture some of the "voices" of women whose culture, language, ethnicity, and class may differ from their own. We must, therefore, be conscious of our Eurocentrism and of how our own biases and experiences color our perceptions of "others."[8] We cannot presume to understand the experiences of different cultures and social groups. Canadian poet and artist Lillian Allen explains: "White writers have to know what they don't know. When you're in a situation of dominance [or power], it's hard for you to know what you don't know."[9]

To address this problem, American historian Gerda Lerner pleads for a new approach to writing history in which "sex, class and race dominance are interrelated and inseparable from the start."[10] She bases her approach on three assumptions:

1. Claims of universality cannot be made from descriptions of the activities of a small elite group of upper-class white females.
2. When we study a group of women, past or present, and make generalizations about them we must take not only the similarities but the differences among them into consideration.
3. We must think not only in terms of priorities or hierarchies of oppression, but also in terms of how one depends on the other.

Lerner reminds us that it is *as* unjust to treat all women (and nurses) as a monolithic group as it has been to subsume all women under the term "men." Differences among women, such as class, ethnicity, culture, religion, and so forth, must be taken into account.

Just what does this mean concretely for the writing of the history of the ICN? It means that we must ask: Does this piece of evidence hold true for women of different ethnicities and classes? And what difference will it make to the whole if we look at the variety of political and cultural contexts in which nursing has flourished (or not flourished)? To answer this, we must focus both on the common core of experiences as well as on the particular in all its variations. We must approach our task by finding new analytic methods that consistently answer the query: Why is this important, and not that? We must ask this question both of ourselves and of the ICN. Why were certain issues important or of interest to the ICN and not others? What interests us as we sift through the data and write the ICN's history?

For example, why was the South African Nursing Association made to answer for their discriminatory policies regarding black nurse participation when other member countries (for example, the United States) had not fully integrated blacks into their national nursing associations?[11] Why were some countries threatened with eviction for unpaid dues when others were not?[12] Why did the ICN champion certain public health initiatives, such as the antismoking campaign, and not others?[13]

Taking these methodological problems and linking them to ICN ideology presents a third dilemma. How do we capture "difference" *among* nurses from a variety of cultures while still explaining the "glue," the "unity," the "sisterhood" that Fenwick wished to create and that has survived the twentieth century? Can we reconcile the tension between cultural hegemony evident in the early ICN leadership and the celebration of national diversity consistently expressed by ICN leaders? If we make difference central to our analysis, we create an interactive contextual model that not only presents different points of view, but also accurately represents the power relations existing among the various groups as they interacted in the same place and time.

Perhaps Mary Adelaide Nutting expressed our tripartite methodological dilemma best. In a poignant 1924 commentary in the ICN publication, *Bulletin,* Nutting broached the subject of organizational integrity.

> If we are to hold together as the professionally trained nurses of the many countries of the world in helpful and strengthening association and good fellowship, we must be able, in the words of England's great prime minister "to differ without being hostile," and to find somewhere between the extremes of thought and opinion the best common working ground.[14]

Unity of Sympathy, Thought, and Purpose

An understanding of Ethel Bedford Fenwick's "international idea" for nurses further exemplifies her push for unity. After attending the International Congress of Women in 1899, Fenwick presented her views to the Matron's Council of Great Britain and Ireland. Fenwick stressed the need for professional education and organization of nurses throughout the world and argued for an international body of nurses to coordinate and implement this agenda.

> If the poet's dream of the brotherhood of man is ever to be fulfilled, then surely a sisterhood of nurses is an international idea, and one in which the women of all nations therefore could be asked and expected to join. The work in which nurses are engaged in other countries is precisely the same as that in our own. . . . We should today here inaugurate an international council of nurses composed of representatives of the nursing councils of every country, a body which shall in the first place help to build up nurses councils in those countries which do not now possess any nursing organization at all, which shall afford to those countries the information acquired in England and America in the progress and development of our work, aiding them with our experiences, helping them to avoid the difficulties which we have met.[15]

Fenwick's argument for worldwide unity of nursing under the purview of American and British know-how may be seen as an example of cultural imperialism characteristic of many other international women's reform organizations during this period.[16] Certainly it corresponds to the evangelistic zeal of women's missionary work and raises further questions. What would non-Western countries have to gain by joining the organization? What did the various countries know and think about themselves and other countries, and did leaders listen? What kinds of generalizations can we make based on what we now know?[17]

Universalizing the "Glue"

Internationalizing Womanhood

We think the first of three transcultural generalizations we can make is that of the common thread of womanhood and nursing's work as expressed by Fenwick in her "international idea." Almost all of the nurses in the ICN were women, and the second phase of the women's movement was an *international* movement.[18] Feminists participated in comparable alliances and organizations such as women's temperance unions, the international alliance for women's suffrage, and the international councils of women.

The ICN supported women's suffrage at its Second Quinquennial Congress held in London in 1909; this stance was of particular importance for unmarried nurses. Lavinia Dock explained, "the industrial spinster does not count. . . . She lives, she works, she disappears; she is a voteless, voiceless item of humanity."[19] The ICN was the voice and vote for many women in a pre–women's suffrage era while its purpose as an "instrument of service to mankind" corresponded to nursing's altruistic service ideal.

Desire for Peace

Second, although many scholars contest the automatic linking of women with peace movements (or with antiwar propaganda), there are many examples of women's international cooperation for peace in the twentieth century. In the United States, the Women's Christian Temperance Union, the Women's Boards of Foreign Missions, and the Young Women's Christian Association (YWCA) were all members of the largest women's peace organization in the 1920s, the National Committee on the Cause and Cure of War.[20]

Indeed, the ICN watchword for 1925, given by President Sophie Mannerheim of Finland, was *peace* and it seems reasonable to assume that the desire for working toward peace in the world must have played some part in the "glue" of the ICN. For well-known American pacifist Lavinia Dock, at least, peace was an important goal. A self-proclaimed "Russian sympathizer" and an active member of the Council of Friendship with Russia, Dock voiced her opinions freely to ICN leaders well into the mid-twentieth century. "Peace," according to Dock, meant the acceptance of competing political ideologies, while "war" was "against opinions, thoughts and ideas" that reflected differences among nations.[21]

However, there are today and have been historically many women's movements and many peace movements in various times and places among different cultures and classes.[22] It is therefore not obvious that women who supported the peace movement were or are "feminist pacifists." For example, for many decades the Women's International League for Peace and Freedom refused to support the American Equal Rights Amendment. Further, we need to know more about the relationship between pacifism and antimilitarism, and what part this played in the ICN sisterhood. Canadian scientist Ursula Franklin points out that "pacifism is not anti-war, pacifism is the advocacy of a way of life in which the roots of war are attacked and war is unnecessary. . . . Pacifism is the wish to eliminate the condition of people being threatened, people being without choice."[23] Pacifism, therefore, is understanding the uses and abuses of *power*. Could this link have been an ideological linchpin for the ICN?

The ICN as Missionary Movement

The last generalization is the role of colonialism in the history of the ICN. Colonialization by the British and Americans, in particular, and the emergence of new cultural and national identities were common themes for many ICN member countries. British imperialistic power alone involved "a quarter of the world's surface and a colonial population of some 400 million people."[24] In fact, of the twenty-one countries that belonged to the ICN before 1930, all were either Anglo or northern European, American or British colonies, or countries influenced by American or British nursing ideologies through the Rockefeller Foundation (see Table 1).

The ICN, in some respects, was a missionary movement whose special mission was to spread American and British nursing culture around the world. Fenwick's appeal to "afford to [other] countries the information acquired in England and America in the progress and development of [nursing] work" embodied the spirit of Anglo North American female moral authority. The presumed advantages for nurses in less advantaged nations were twofold: the position of nursing and women's status would be improved and nursing in other countries would be exposed to superior Western nursing knowledge.[25]

The Philippines is an interesting example of the spread of Western imperialism. An American colony after its "liberation" from Spanish rule in 1898, the Philippine islands became a special project of the Rockefeller Foundation in the 1920s. On the recommendation of Dr. Victor G. Heiser, who surveyed the public health conditions in the Philippines in 1921, the Rockefeller Foundation agreed to finance, among other things, public health nursing training.[26] Alice Fitzgerald was appointed the nurse consultant to introduce public health nursing to Philippine hospital nursing schools. The former director of the division of nurses of the League of Red Cross Societies, Fitzgerald had served with the American Red Cross throughout western and eastern Europe.[27] Beginning her two-year assignment in April 1922, Fitzgerald listed among her objectives a plan to organize a National Nursing Organization for the Philippine islands to "stimulate professional esprit de corps."[28] Six months after her arrival in September

Table 1. ICN Membership by Country and Year of Admission.

1904	*1922*
Germany* (1949)	Belgium
United Kingdom	Italy* (1949)
United States	Norway
1909	*1925*
Canada	France
Denmark	Ireland
Finland	Poland* (1961)
Netherlands	
	1929
1912	Australia
India	Brazil
New Zealand	Greece
	Philippines
	Sweden
	Yugoslavia* (1957)

Compiled from *International Nursing Review* 21 (May–August, 1974): 79, and Sheila Quinn, *ICN: Past and Present* (ICN: Scutari Press, 1989): 211.
*Countries were originally accepted into the ICN and then readmitted after membership lapsed.
See Winifred Hector, *The Work of Mrs. Bedford Fenwick and the Rise of Professional Nursing* (University of London, 1970), 50. "The first half of the twentieth century was dislocated by two World conflicts. . . . The ICN list of its member countries reflects not only the fortunes of nursing in these countries but their political histories."

1922, the Filipino Nurses Associaation (FNA) was formed. By 1929 the FNA had joined the ICN.

Suppressing Political Difference

We argue that the ICN used professional ideology to overcome class, ethnic, and cultural differences. A professionalist stance provided a means of neutral, "apolitical" control that supported the model of "unity." The emphasis on the "nonpolitical" and "nonsectarian" is a most interesting theme that requires further analysis. The idea stipulated that women/nurses should band together in the interest of humanity rather than their own self-interest. As Fenwick put it, "We nurses, unlike the members of many other professions, are happily untroubled by national considerations. . . . our work stands apart from every influence excepting that which permits the health, and therefore in a huge measure the happiness, of the peoples of the world."[29]

By maintaining political neutrality, the ICN could achieve internal cohesion while assuring the public that they, as women, were not engaged in party politics. "To introduce party politics into nursing," wrote Bertha Wellin, was to "degrade the spirit of [nursing] service in the professional spirit and undermine the good fellowship which latter for the majority of nurses replaced homelife."[30] Could unity have meant the suppression of difference rather than the integration of variance? Perhaps unity through the common rhetoric of nurses work was the "glue" that held the ICN together in the first three decades.

Making Difference Central

Using Gerda Lerner's assumptions about writing international history, we conclude our discussion by contemplating approaches to the task ahead. What must be done to account for difference?

First, we must dismantle, historicize, and deconstruct previous meanings and descriptions of the activities of the ICN as defined through the small elite group of ICN nursing leaders.[31] Otherwise we simply create a Western, Eurocentric version of the organization. One way to avoid this trap is to learn as much as possible from historians of nursing from the various ICN participant countries. We have asked every ICN participant nation to provide us with their nursing histories (if available) and/or to give us names of individuals with whom we can consult regarding their particular histories. This will help us situate the various phenomena in their suitable cultural contexts. We seem to have an idea of "the common" through the ICN minutes. However, we must tease out "the difference"—those values, ideas and thoughts that may conflict with the expressed "agreements." We must seek out primary sources as a way to resist overdependence on secondary sources or primary sources that reflect the thoughts and ideas only of the ICN leaders.

Just as Ethel Fenwick judged non-Western countries for their lack of "progress and development," we must be careful to avoid (unwittingly) leaving out cultural differences in the name of writing a "unified" history of the ICN. Those nurses who were colonized, or those who lacked access to so-called civilization and scientific knowledge, have been misrepresented as backward and nonprogressive.[32] In effect, their lack of access may have allowed them to discover innovative ways of caring for people about which Westerners knew nothing. Thus we realize that it is important in revision history to consider knowledge from the margins and not just from the center. As historian Nancy Hewitt points out:

> It is not the center that determines the periphery but the periphery that [in its boundedness] determines the center. Critical dimensions of experience are illuminated by comparison of the margins with the center.[33]

Challenging Dichotomies

In the first three decades of the twentieth century, the ICN's considerable attention to political neutrality may have helped maintain unity amidst difference. Further, unity may have suppressed difference by minimizing the political and national differences among the organization's membership, or it may have represented a collection of principally white Anglo-European voices and ideas.

Many countries and nurses who made up the core of the ICN were marginalized even as they were accepted as members "in a confederation of workers" to advance "greater unity of thought, sympathy and purpose."[34] Part of our task must be to acknowledge the "other" as equally important or perhaps as even more important in our analysis than have previous historical analyses of the ICN. Only by focusing equally on the experiences of women who were among the colonized can we "reveal the ways that female colonizers reinforced, even as they resisted, imperialistic designs."[35]

Barbara L. Brush
Research Associate, ICN Centennial History Project
Doctoral Candidate, School of Nursing, University of Pennsylvania
8629 Patton Road
Wyndmoor, Pa. 19118
Phone: (215) 836-1285

Meryn Stuart
Project Historian, ICN Centennial History Project
Assistant Professor, School of Nursing
Adjunct Hannah Professor, History of Medicine, Faculty of Medicine
University of Ottawa
RR # 1 Box 123
McDonald's Corners
Ontario, Canada K0G1M0
Phone: (613) 278-2373

Acknowledgments

The authors wish to acknowledge the support of the International Council of Nurses and the Rockefeller Foundation in the preparation of this manuscript.

Notes

1. The establishment of the ICN followed on the heels of the organization of the International Council of Women (ICW). The first ICW conference was held in Washington, D.C., in 1888, with forty-nine women from eleven countries in attendance. Fenwick attended the second conference in 1898 and shortly thereafter proposed her "international idea" for nurses.

2. Sheila Quinn estimated that 1.2 million nurses were represented by 100 member countries in 1988. See Dame Sheila Quinn, *ICN Past and Present* (Scutari Press, 1989), xi.

3. This project is supported by a grant from the ICN. Joan Lynaugh of the University of Pennsylvania, U.S.A., heads a team including: Meryn Stuart from the University of Ottawa, Canada; Anne Marie Rafferty from the University of Nottingham, England; Nancy Tomes from the State University of New York at Stony Brook, U.S.A.; and Barbara Brush from the University of Pennsylvania.

4. We focus our discussion on the first three decades both for the sake of brevity and because we believe the years between 1899 and 1930 reflect the ICN's most critical period of development as an international women's organization.

5. For a discussion of these differing contexts, see Karen Offen, Ruth R. Pierson, and Jane Rendall, eds., "Introduction," in *Writing Women's History: International Perspectives* (Bloomington and Indianapolis: Indiana University Press, 1991), xix–xli.

6. Judith Allen, "Contextualizing Late Nineteenth Century Feminism: Problems and Comparisons" (Paper presented at the Conference of the Canadian Historical Association, University of Victoria, British Columbia), 18 and 19 May 1990.

7. Ibid.

8. Gerda Lerner, "Reconceptualizing Differences Among Women," *Journal of Women's History* 3 (Winter 1990): 106–22. Lerner discusses the use of the term "other" as a negative "mark" that is applied by dominant groups.

9. Quoted by Ruth Roach Pierson, "Experience, Difference, Dominance and Voice in the Writing of Canadian Women's History," in Offer, Pierson, and Rendell, *Writing Women's History,* 90.

10. Lerner, 110.

11. Grand Council, Minutes of Meetings, 27, 28, 29 May and 1 June 1957, Rome, Italy, Annex VIII, pp. 35–51, ICN Archives, Geneva, Switzerland (hereafter cited as ICNA). South Africa was accused of racial discrimination, allowing European nurses but not native nurses to join in national nursing membership. This practice was in conflict with ICN's code of ethics.

12. Dues payment was often a source of controversy. In the first thirty-year period, an interesting discussion of the German Nurses Association's lack of dues

payment in the minutes exemplifies the dilemma of whether countries who did not pay should be allowed to remain in the ICN. See Minutes of the Meeting of the Board of Directors, Report of the Standing Committee on Finance, 29 June–1 July 1931, Geneva, Switzerland, pp. 29–33, ICNA.

13. The ICN's 1973 pledge to support the World Health Organization's "Limitation of Smoking" campaign represents the organization's first health policy stance. See ICN Minutes of the Meeting of the Board of Directors, Report of the Professional Services Committee to the Council of National Representatives, May 1973, Mexico City, p. 10, ICNA.

14. M. Adelaide Nutting, Chairman of the Committee on Education, *Bulletin IV* (October 1924), p. 2, ICNA.

15. Ethel Bedford Fenwick, Address to Matron's Council Conference, 1 July 1899, ICN Minutes, ICNA.

16. Our definition of imperialism is taken from Nupur Chaudhuri and Margaret Strobel, eds., *Western Women and Imperialism: Complicity and Resistance* (Bloomington: Indiana University Press, 1992), 2. "Imperialism is a concept that signifies any relationship of dominance and subordination between nations."

17. For further discussion of these issues, see Thomas G. Paterson, "A Round Table: Explaining the History of American Foreign Relations," *The Journal of American History* (June 1990): 90.

18. See Allen, 3, and Carol Miller, "Lobbying the League: Women's International Organizations and the League of Nations" (Doctoral thesis, Oxford University, 1992). Miller argues that women's organizations were divided into four categories: feminist, professional, religious, and pacifist. While they had distinct goals and priorities, all aimed to advance the status of women.

19. Lavinia Dock, "Foreign Delegates and Organizations," *American Journal of Nursing* 1 (September 1901): 864–65.

20. Susan Ziegler, "Finding a Cure for War: Women's Politics and the Peace Movement in the 1920s," *Journal of Social History* 24, no. 1 (Fall 1990): 69–86. See note 18.

21. Dock readily blamed the United States for the poor relations with Russia after World War II. She strongly urged the ICN to encourage membership by the Russian nurses, who to this day are not members. Lavinia Dock to Princess Anna Schwarzenberg, 18 March 1947, 17 May 1947, Lavinia Dock Correspondence 1947–1951, ICNA; Lavinia Dock to Gerda Hojer, 19 July 1947, ICNA.

22. For a discussion of the relationship between feminism and pacifism, see Berenice Carroll, "Feminism and Pacifism: Historical and Theoretical Connections," in *Women and Peace. Theoretical and Practical Perspectives,* ed. Ruth R. Pierson (London: Croom Helm, 1987), 2–28.

23. Commentary by Ursula Franklin on Berenice Carroll (above) in Pierson, *Women and Peace,* 24.

24. Paul Thompson, *The Voice of the Past,* 2nd ed. (Oxford: Oxford University Press, 1988), 84.

25. See Patricia R. Hill, *The World Their Household: The American Women's Foreign Mission Movement and Cultural Transformation, 1870–1920* (Ann Arbor: University of Michigan Press, 1985). Hill examines the cultural and ideological climate

of foreign missions and women's evangelizing work. As evangelism broadened to include social service, preachers were replaced by nurses, teachers, and social workers who had "considerable interest in the spread of American culture" (p. 130).

26. Minutes of the International Health Board, 16 December 1921, RG 1.1, Project Series 242C *Philippines,* Folder 47, Rockefeller Archive Center, North Tarrytown, New York (hereafter cited as RAC).

27. Minutes of the International Health Board, 24 October 1922, RG 1.1, Project Series 242C *Philippines,* Folder 47, RAC. Fitzgerald served in France, Italy, Poland, Czechoslovakia, Serbia, Albania, Montenegro, Salaniki, and Romania.

28. Alice Fitzgerald to Victor G. Heiser, 22 May 1922, RG 1.1, Project Series 242C *Philippines,* Folder 47, RAC.

29. Ethel Bedford Fenwick, Address of Welcome, Minutes of the Second Quinquennial Meeting, 19 July 1909, United Kingdom, ICNA.

30. Bertha Wellin, "Politics and Nurses" (Editorial), *The ICN* 2 (January 1927): 2.

31. Previous histories of the ICN were written by those who were part of the small group of leaders. In light of new social historical methods, we may suggest different interpretations of many of the same events and activities of the ICN. However, the earlier work is invaluable in helping us to understand much of the ICN's workings and activities. See Daisy Bridges, *A History of the ICN 1899–1964: The First Sixty-Five Years* (Philadelphia, Pa.: J. B. Lippincott Co., 1967), and Quinn, *ICN Past and Present.*

32. For a fascinating analysis of the concept of "civilization" and how one African-American woman subverted dominant discourses in the late nineteenth century, see Gail Bederman, "'Civilization,' the Decline of Middle-Class Manliness and Ida B. Well's Antilynching Campaign (1892–94)," *Radical History Review* 52 (1992): 5–32.

33. Nancy Hewitt, "Reflections from a Departing Editor: Recasting Issues of Marginality," *Gender and History* (Spring 1991): 5.

34. ICN Constitution, Preamble, July 1990, ICN minutes, ICNA.

35. Hewitt, 4.

BOOK REVIEWS

Yellow Fever and Public Health in the New South

By John H. Ellis
(Lexington: University of Kentucky, 1992)

The study of epidemics has enticed historians for centuries. Following in the tradition of William McNeill's seminal work *Plagues and People* (1976), John Ellis traces changes in society following the yellow fever epidemic of 1878 in the southern United States. More specifically, Ellis identifies the birth of the public health movement in the new South as one of the significant outcomes of a virulent and devastating epidemic that caused 20,000 deaths and financial losses of almost 200 million dollars in the lower Mississippi Valley. Focusing on three major cities—New Orleans, Memphis, and Atlanta, the commercial and economic leaders of the post–Civil War South—he links the growth of the cities to the steadily deteriorating environmental conditions in which their inhabitants lived and worked.

In the preface Ellis introduces the major themes of the book. The first theme focuses on the complacency of the cities' "comfortable class" residents who accepted as inevitable the high rates of disease and death in the poor and immigrant classes. The poor, it was believed, were often ill and died because of their immoral, lazy, and criminal behaviors. Ellis documents that this sense of complacency of the upper classes would be threatened and then shattered by the lethal epidemics of the 1870s that indiscriminately invaded their businesses and homes.

Responding, at times reluctantly, to the developing knowledge that there was a relationship between disease, mortality, and poor sanitary conditions of the city and their own health and happiness, the "comfortable class" eventually lent some support to the establishment of municipal boards of health in the 1850s. These municipal boards would, through the valiant efforts of a few enlightened civic and physician leaders, attempt to protect the health of the community by instituting some control over the quality of the cities' food, water, and drainage disposal.

A second theme of the book involves disputes among physicians of the era as to the etiology of infectious disease. The physicians' lack of scientific knowledge as to the cause of the epidemics unfortunately limited their ability both to advise civil authorities on how to protect citizens and to effectively treat the thousands of victims of the pestilence.

The most prevalent theories of the causation of disease during the era included those of the contagionists, anticontagionists, and the contingent-contagionists. Contagionists believed that specific entities, or contagia, caused disease. Proponents of the anticontagionist theory believed that disease, especially in epidemic proportions, was attributed to miasma, an infected state of the atmosphere that induced human disease. The third group, the contingent-contagionists, assumed a more eclectic view of disease. They believed in both the power of specific and nonspecific contagia and the need of specific atmospheric, environmental, and social conditions. Lacking a uniform understanding of disease, and thus a unified voice, physicians' actions and advice were often at odds with one another. At the zenith of human misery and destruction during the 1878 epidemic, all three views competed with superstition and witchcraft to stem the fear and death engulfing the communities.

Ellis's final theme focuses on the personal, political, and economic needs of people and cities that complicate the health measures taken to stop the spread of the epidemics. Often these needs are in conflict. Responding to the fear of the spread of disease, quarantine procedures were established in many areas surrounding the plague zone to prevent, sometimes with the use of guns, the entrance of people or goods from the epidemic communities. People's inability to find refuge from the epidemic plus the interruption of commerce between cities added and extended the human misery.

In chapter 1, Ellis traces the physical, economic, and social growth of the cities and their early efforts, in the 1850s, to address the need for adequate municipal sanitation. Corruption and lack of public support for the legislative authority to force compliance of the rudimentary sanitary measures undertaken left New Orleans, and its sister river city Memphis, particularly vulnerable to the frequent epidemics of Asiatic cholera and yellow fever that began to appear in the 1830s. For decades these epidemics struck almost exclusively among the poor and immigrant class of the cities and towns along the Mississippi River, leading the comfortable class to believe that the epidemics were "strangers' diseases."

Despite its fortunate exemption from the ravages of cholera and yellow fever epidemics, Atlanta had a fearful mortality rate resulting from poor sanitation, which qualified it to be included in the area Ellis labels the Necropolitan South. Lacking an accurate record of the three cities' mortality rates over the years, a conservative estimate for the period of 1855–60 places the "annual average mortality rate of New Orleans at slightly over forty-five per thousand," that of Memphis "at about forty," and that of Atlanta "at slightly under thirty." Considering that the nation's overall death rate at the time was "between twenty-one and twenty-three per thousand," the three cities' excess is awesome (p. 33).

Searching for answers to why the South's public health movement, in spite of frequent epidemics, failed to move as quickly to gain acceptance as in the North, Ellis argues that the culture of the area bred indifference and antipathy to such activity. "Within the context of a southern slaveholding society, a society ruled by the paternal authority of a slaveholding class, assertion of liberal, urban bourgeois values, such as sanitary reform, were anathema to the governing ideology" (p. 35). This attitude was also sustained for decades by the erroneous notion that native-born city residents, especially of the middle and upper classes, possessed an innate or acquired immunity to the epidemic diseases.

Yellow fever, originally brought to the Western Hemisphere by the African slave trade, was, in May of 1878, not a new disease when a crewman from a ship from Havana died in New Orleans of fever. The story of the spread of an especially virulent form of yellow fever, not only in New Orleans and Memphis but throughout the lower Mississippi Valley, constitutes the second chapter of the book. It is a story of panic as thousands of middle-class families, after death had claimed many of their children, fled the cities; of the courage of those who remained behind to offer relief to the stricken; and of the drunkenness and greed of some who preyed upon the sick and plundered the unprotected cities and towns.

The accounts of the physician, religious, and lay volunteers struggling to minister to the thousands of sick and dying are the most touching portions of the book. Under staggering conditions, many contracted the disease and significant numbers died. While the discussion of the role of nursing during the epidemics is quite brief, the contributions of Catholic and Episcopal nuns and community women are particularly acknowledged. These women gave unstintingly of themselves in the care of the sick. Not all women however, were altruistic. A Memphis physician wrote that "while many excellent and worthy nurses came [to help], others also came whose only purpose seemed to be plunder and the gratification of alcoholic thirst, and whose presence here was scarcely less destructive to human life then the plague itself" (p. 50).

The quest for health reform and its necessary legislation comprises the remaining chapters of the book. The response of the nation to the plight of the southern plague victims, and the government's realization that the development of a national transportation system now left even distant communities vulnerable to epidemics, sparked a public debate as to whether the federal government or the individual states should be responsible for the protection of citizens. The long, personal, and destructive contest between two of the early leaders of American public health, Dr. John Woolsworth, surgeon general of the U.S. Marine Hospital, and Dr. John Shaw Billings, vice president of the American Public Health Association, over the leadership of a proposed national sanitary bureau supports Ellis's thesis that public health reform was a highly politicized process. At stake were not only different theories as to the etiology of disease but also fear among state authorities about the growing power of the federal government to control interstate commerce, especially through the use of embargoes against goods leaving epidemic areas. The combined strength of city business leaders with railroad and industrial corporations, whose economic status was threatened by proposed federal actions, tipped the scale in favor of the rights of states to manage their own boards of health. As Ellis notes, "only in later times, and under different political circumstances, would the idea of a strong federal agency having broad responsibility for public health receive national acceptance" (p. 82).

Left to their own initiative, public health reform measures were instituted in the South, led notably by Memphis and New Orleans. Efforts were made to drain wetlands, construct sewer systems, protect the quality of food and water consumed by citizens, and isolate, through quarantine, infected individuals. The South's lack of economic resources to pay for these health services, however, restricted the full development of a public health system. The significance of the 1878 yellow fever epidemic, in Ellis's opinion, was that it served as a significant force in shaping both the South's and the nation's public health movements.

To those currently advocating more emphasis on preventive health versus acute care medicine, the reading of this book will warn of the power of economic interest groups. It is a legitimate warning. To expect groups—physicians, businesses, and so forth—whose livelihood depends on the current system to expire voluntarily in the cause of the general welfare of the community is as naive now as it was in the 1880s. Others who may enjoy and benefit from reading this book are those interested in the history of public health at both the state and national levels. Public health medicine is by far the most political form of health care in the country. Although public health medicine's ability to protect the health and welfare of citizens has been proven many times, public health officials face a continuous battle to obtain and direct the necessary resources to ensure a quality of life for all citizens. John Ellis's study of the yellow fever epidemic of 1878 captures this continuing dilemma.

Barbara Brodie, PhD, RN
Professor
School of Nursing
University of Virginia
Charlottesville, Va.

Framing Disease: Studies in Cultural History

Ed. by Charles Rosenberg and Janet Golden
(New Brunswick, N.J.: Rutgers University Press, 1992)

Each piece in this extraordinary rich collection illustrates that "disease" is a biological event with social implications. Written from a cultural history perspective, each essay highlights the power of disease as a fundamental social problem, as a creator of institutions and organized work, as an impetus for social policy, and as a prism through which major cultural issues are refracted. As Charles Rosenberg (1989) observes, "in some ways, disease does not exist until we have agreed that it does, by perceiving, naming, and responding to it." Once extant, disease becomes simultaneously an elusive entity and a powerful reality with economic, social, legal, philosophical, and historical implications.

Rosenberg's learned introduction argues that while the social-constructionist viewpoint of disease origin has successfully reminded us that medical thought and practice are culturally dependent, the perspective has overemphasized functionalist ends. Rosenberg persuades the reader that historians have slighted the connection between the biological and social aspects of disease and uses the metaphor of "framing," fashioned from Erving Goffman's work (1974, 1972), to emphasize that biology often shapes the choices available in conceptualizing, experiencing, and legitimizing disease.

Framing disease, according to Rosenberg, is a process that inevitably begins with questions regarding how and why ailments originate. The answers are, of course, dependent on the existing theories that have included, for example, the eighteenth-century theory of humoral balance, the nineteenth-century idea of environmental contamination by germs, and the twentieth-century autoimmune-genetic explanations. Once "framed" by the era's thought style, symptoms of specific illnesses become categorized and accepted and the disease becomes an acknowledged actor in a complex set of social negotiations between the experts, the laymen, and the social institutions concerned with disease. Disease, as such, shapes life-styles, creates business markets, produces institutions, and molds reality in very sobering ways. Rosenberg subtly suggests an inverse relationship between a disease's circumference and the individual's "self." That is, episodic acute disease influences a patient's regime and lifestyle, but chronic disease engulfs the patient and, in very significant ways, *becomes* the patient's life. The perception of time, the quality of relationships, bodily functions, and "being" are mediated by chronic diseases such as schizophrenia, cancer, and AIDS.

Four essays of this collection explore how evolving frameworks of pathological assumptions define and redefine disease and its treatment. Case studies of kidney disease (Steven Peitzman); rheumatic fever (Peter English); parasitology (John Farley); and coronary thrombosis (Christopher Lawrence) provide illuminating accounts of the complex process of how diseases come to be identified and how the sociological, empirical, and epistemological twists have shaped the current form of understanding each disease. As accepted biological "facts" change, the possible explanations of disease alter, creating dynamic and nonlinear shifts in medical thought and treatment. Scientists and physicians, called the "would-be-farmers" by Rosenberg, negotiate the mélange of knowledge, hoping to locate a unified understanding of the disease, while at the same time using the changing theories to define themselves as experts.

Another four essays focus explicitly on disease as a "frame"—where disease serves as a structuring factor for people's lives. As Rosenberg observes, one of the most striking aspects of the interaction between medicine and society in the late nineteenth century was the tendency to medicalize deviance. Attached to changing cultural, intellectual, and intrapsychic contexts, the boundaries between sin and illness shifted. Behavior once identified as aberrant now was identified as illness. Case studies of suicide (Michael MacDonald), homosexuality (Bert Hansen), anorexia nervosa (Joan Jacobs Brumberg), and chronic fatigue syndrome (Robert Aronowitz) collectively illustrate how disease entities, based on behavior, emerged. Once visible, diseases became an emotional option for persons and provided an explanatory framework of identity to otherwise unfathomable behavior. Moreover, as aberrant behaviors are relabeled "disease," medical specialities, subcultures, and institutions are created around the disease so as to reinforce its reality, to manage its stigmatization, and to establish focal points of interaction.

Disease also enters the public domain. In the arena of the public's health, disease becomes an object of debate, negotiation, and power strategies. Negotiators in the public arena include unions, insurance companies, reformers, and government officials who create policies and make judgments. Two essays consider how diseases are negotiated in the public arena by examining the politics of silicosis (Gerald Markowitz and David Rosner) and the legality of psychiatric diagnoses (Janet Tighe), while a third essay (John Eyler) presents an enlightening view of the transgenerational debate regarding social responsibility for the sick poor. The authors articulate how law, business, science, and medicine express different needs and perspectives in framing disease and, subsequently, advocate disparate views in determining right from wrong, individual from collective responsibility, and reasoned argument from emotional rationale.

Beyond the cultural dialogues, intellectual negotiations, and political duels that surround disease, institutions are constructed to manage disease and to care for the victims of disease. Barbara Bates fashions an empathetic story of the care of consumptives in Pennsylvania, emphasizing the bargains crafted between patients and caretakers to manage sickness, instill hope, and rationalize prolonged dependency; Ellen Dwyer creates a graceful portrayal of one institution's efforts to mediate between perspectives of lay persons, experts, and intellectuals in caring for epileptic patients. An insightful essay by Elizabeth Fee ends the collection with a discussion of Henry Sigerist's vision of physicians' dual role as social advocates in the "people's war for health" and as providers of individualized care. Fee's essay bestows an artful unity to the book's theme, which escorts the reader full circle to rereading the introduction.

This book is a splendid collection of work that, using the metaphor of framing, examines the intricacy of disease as a complex phenomenon that defines boundaries within cultures. The essays are sculpted by seasoned historians skilled in interpreting the nuances and subtle meanings of cultural history.

History, like all disciplines, is itself a social system and presupposes a sociology of thinking or a culture of inquiry. Rosenberg seems to be shepherding historians away from the "social constructionist" approach and widening the perspective by using Goffman's sociological "frame" perspective, which was, in turn, borrowed from Gregory Bateson (1955). The frame metaphor does encourage, in the spirit of Fleck (1979) and LaTour and Woolgar (1979), a comparative epistemological perspective that promotes the "insights-become-concepts" process. Even more enticing is that the frame metaphor highlights the recurring thorny issue regarding the power of institutions to reduce the "self" to an object that occupies no social space. If thinking is "framed" by institutions, what is the historian to do with the concepts of the "I," the "person," the "me," and the "self"? Of course, for generations many able thinkers like Emile Durkheim and Robert Merton have wrestled with the question and have speculated on the relationship between the individual mind and social influences on cognition. The idea of "frame" encourages historians to inquire how perceptions and ideas from the lived experiences of "I" (or diseased individuals) may modify both the "experts'" and the institutions' thinking, their definitions of knowledge, and their perception of reality. In particular, Aronowitz's essay on chronic fatigue syndrome and Bates's piece on tuberculosis begin to explore the juncture and mechanisms by which the patients' thinking and lived experience of disease inform and define clinical practice.

The collection will appeal to a wide range of readers, including health care professionals curious about the history of disease, as well as historians (social, cultural, intellectual) committed to researching health and illness within society. From a pedagogical perspective, the essays could be assigned to undergraduate students interested in the description of disease formulation, as well as to doctoral students exploring critical thinking and the sociology of knowledge. The essays are a "good fireside read," as well as intellectually provocative and challenging.

In some ways, nurses may experience this book as challenging. Much like the work of Koffka or Kierkegaard, Rosenberg's insightful piercing commentary provides a scholarly but brusque backdrop for the essays, leaving the reader with neither doubts of physicians' cultural authority nor uncertainty regarding the vulnerability of an individual patient. Interestingly, nurses are rendered nebulous by the authors. This impalpable view of nurses in the "history of disease" could be construed as a sad commentary on nursing. On the other hand, the essays' portrayal of nurses as obscure may, in fact, be one of the more fascinating questions for the nursing discipline. By necessity, nursing is often placed in what Engelhardt (1982) called the "in-between." That is, the nurse exists between the patient and the physician, between the institution and the patient, between the institution and the physician, between competing frames, and lastly, between the patient and the disease. As Rosenberg suggests, "we see . . . what we have been prepared to see" (p. 186). Although historians may find the in-between position of nursing difficult to visualize, nurses believe that this in-between position is not synonymous with "invisible." Still, from the historical and current-day perspectives, both the significance and meaning of nursing within the complex context of disease remain unclear. Rosenberg and Golden have, as one would anticipate, created another historical work that encourages mental aerobics. The book forces on the reader unasked questions, challenges old perspectives, demands cognitive flexibility, and makes the ordinary quite sublime.

DIANE HAMILTON, PhD, RN
Assistant Professor
School of Nursing
University of Rochester
Rochester, N.Y.

References

Bateson, Gregory. "A Theory of Play and Phantasy." *Psychological Research Reports* 2 (December 1955): 39–51.
Engelhardt, Tristan. "Illnesses, Diseases, and Sickness." In *The Humanity of the Ill*, ed. Vern Kestenbaum (Knoxville: University of Tennessee Press, 1982), 142–86.
Fleck, Ludwig. *The Genesis of a Scientific Fact* (Chicago: University of Chicago Press, 1979).
Goffman, Erving. *Frame Analysis: An Essay on the Organization of Experience* (Cambridge: Harvard University Press, 1974).
———. *Steps to an Ecology of the Mind* (New York: Ballantine Books, 1972).
LaTour, Bruno, and Steven Woolgar. *Laboratory Life* (Beverly Hills: Sage, 1979).
Rosenberg, Charles. "Disease in History: Frames and Framers." *Milbank Quarterly*, 67 (suppl. 1, 1989): 1–15.

First Words: Selected Addresses from the National League for Nursing, 1894–1933

Ed. by Nettie Birnbach and Sandra Lewenson
(New York: National League for Nursing Press, 1991)

Reading the articles in this book is almost like a walk through history. Early nursing leaders—Adelaide Nutting, Isabel Hampton Robb, Annie Goodrich, Lavinia Dock, Effie Taylor, Lillian Wald—are all represented, as well as others who are less well known.

As the subtitle suggests, the editors have included published speeches presented at national meetings of the organizations that were forerunners of the present National League for Nursing. Technically, the subtitle is a misnomer, since the National League for Nursing dates to 1952, but one can understand the editors' dilemma in including in the title the American Society of Superintendents of Training Schools for Nurses (1893–1912) and the National League of Nursing Education (1912–1952). The history of these name changes is explained in both the preface and the forward to the book.

The book is divided into six sections, with addresses presented chronologically in each. These six sections address the following areas: education, control of practice, recruitment, ethics, image, and power. This division contributes to the ease in using the book; for instance, should one wish to explore the background of current concerns about the image of nursing, one need only to refer to that section.

Articles were selected with care, and each one contributes to the particular section in which it is located. This reviewer found the sections on image and power especially interesting. The use of these particular words is relatively recent in discussing these two concepts; nonetheless, the articles reflect the authors' concerns about what today is called the image of nursing, and their ideas about what can be done to improve it. Early nursing leaders were well aware of the need to overcome the poor image portrayed by the unskilled, inept, and sometimes corrupt workers who were the predecessors of trained nurses. They recognized that the delivery of high quality care was required to assure public support of nursing, and directed a great deal of attention to educating nurses whose competency could positively change the image of nursing.

In the section on power, the term *power* is recognized and explored in relation to the nursing profession. Sophie Palmer discusses "The Power of the Professional Press," and Sara Parsons explores the power of the superintendent of nurses. Several of the essays identify the role of professional organizations and unified efforts in achieving power. The strongly worded 1910 resolution on the authority of nurses for nursing may surprise some readers by its intensity (pp. 322–23).

Early concerns about ethics were sometimes confused with what might be better termed professional etiquette, and may seem a far cry from the ethical dilemmas facing nurses today. By today's standards, some of the topics covered seem somewhat superficial, yet the articles reflect a concern about ethical issues from the beginning of organized nursing. The Code for Professional Nurses became a reality after the time period covered in this book, but the need for such a code of ethics is identified in several of the articles.

This book is an important contribution to the nursing literature. Many aspects of nursing history that are unfamiliar—perhaps unbelievable—to students and young practitioners are found in the speeches of the time. Anna Alline's description of students' experiences in 1907 was no exaggeration: "Seven days a week . . . fifty weeks a year . . . six to nine months . . . on night duty, and the nights are twelve hours long, eighty-four hours a week" (p. 155).

Some of the essays provide a backdrop for the development of an individual's professional thought. For example, in her 1933 address, Shirley Titus, then dean of the School of Nursing at Vanderbilt University, clearly demonstrates her dissatisfaction with the current system of nursing education and its "social ineffectualness." She decries the organization of schools of nursing as integral parts of hospitals and calls for an entirely new curriculum to meet the changing needs of society, including a plea for state support of nursing education. Did this dissatisfaction lead to her changing her professional role as educator to that of administrator of a state nurses' association, and becoming a pioneer and outspoken advocate for a strong economic security program for nurses?

The source for each article is listed in the references. For those instances in which a speaker in a given essay refers to a speech presented at the same convention but not included in this volume, additional reference notes would be helpful. For example, when Annie Goodrich refers in her address to "those matters which Mrs. Burgess has so ably presented," it would be enlightening to know which matters were presented (p. 283). Later when she refers to "that kind of joyous service Dr. (Glenn) Frank discussed," a little more information about that joyous service would have been helpful (p. 285).

Certainly this book is not intended as historiography, and in many instances readers will need to refer to other sources to fully appreciate the editors' point of view. While the commentary before each section adds an important dimension in this regard, content occasionally called for an explanation that could easily have been footnoted. For example, in her 1911 essay on the University of Minnesota School of Nursing Louise Powell writes, "To the credit of Dr. Board"; it would have been useful to know that this referred to Dr. Richard Olding Beard, credited with founding the University of Minnesota School of Nursing (p. 162). The typographical error was no doubt in the original league report, but a brief acknowledgment and explanation would have underscored the significance of the content.

And for those who might not have known that Isabel Hampton and Mrs. Hunter Robb were the same person, a footnote explanation would have been useful. In fact, two of the addresses in the table of contents are listed as presented by Hunter Robb, when in reality they should have been listed as Mrs. Hunter Robb (Isabel Hampton Robb).

First Words cannot be used as a substitute for the published reports of the annual conventions, but since those documents are frequently difficult to locate, it provides easy access to many of the ideas of the early nursing leaders. Thus, it is a most useful resource for nursing historians and others interested in the development of the profession and in the study of women's issues. Lavinia Dock's words, "Women who nurse ought to be paid equally with men who nurse," remind us that nursing was in the forefront of some of the issues that continue to confront women (p. 89).

Nurse educators will find the book a useful supplement not only in teaching nursing history but also in providing background to investigating contemporary nursing issues. It documents the struggles of early nursing leaders with some concerns that are still unresolved, and it may raise questions about why they are still unresolved.

The editors have done well to include as an epilogue Adelaide Nutting's "Thirty Years of Progress in Nursing" (1923). This period saw a remarkable growth in the numbers of schools of nursing and the numbers of nurses; it witnessed the expansion of fields of nursing, the development of nursing organizations, the creation of nurse practice acts, and the beginnings of a literature of nursing. It also saw significant changes in nursing education, including the development of collegiate schools of nursing. Nutting's paper demonstrates that, in the concluding words of the editors, "The first 40 years left a legacy that changed the profession and had a profound impact on health care in America."

SIGNE COOPER, RN, MEd, FAAN
Professor Emeritus, UW-Madison School of Nursing
Continuing Education in Nursing
Madison, Wis.

Natural Allies: Women's Associations in American History

By Anne Firor Scott
(Urbana and Chicago: University of Illinois Press, 1991)

It was historian Mary Ritter Beard who first attempted to document the essential role American women have played in the building and maintenance of communities. Her 1915 survey, *Women's Work in Municipalities,* commissioned by the National Municipal League, described thousands of municipal reforms and community improvements carried out by various organizations of women. Though criticized by later historians for being light on scholarly documentation and perhaps misleadingly positive in its emphasis on successes, the book at least did call attention to a neglected part of women's history.

In spite of this and other historical efforts by Beard, however, women's contributions were again relegated to a scholarly limbo. It wasn't until the 1970s that release came at the hands of feminism's "second wave" historians.

Anne Firor Scott was one of the first of this group to seriously examine the achievements of "women's clubs." It was in researching what has become a classic, *The Southern Lady: From Pedestal to Politics, 1830–1930* (Chicago: University of Chicago Press, 1970), that Scott discovered women "in their missionary societies, temperance organizations, and literary societies remaking the social and political landscapes of the early-twentieth-century South" and found herself puzzled that "this activity had never found its way into any of the standard histories." This discovery led to new work, and in a real sense the resultant study, *Natural Allies: Women's Associations in American History,* completes with scholarly thoroughness and grace the work begun by Beard some seventy-five years earlier. (In fact, Scott summarizes Beard's data in an appendix.) In these pages Scott demonstrates that not only have women's organizations been ubiquitous; they have been central to American social and political development.

The subject, Scott acknowledges, is complex, and would be made easier "if women had moved in lockstep through stages of development from religious societies to self-improvement clubs, to civic improvement, to suffrage and so on. But no such tidy order emerges from the record. Groups with different purposes emerged at the same time, and what is more confusing, their boundaries were anything but fixed." (For example, not all women's reform groups supported suffrage, and some women who worked together on various reforms disagreed as to the desirability of women's voting rights.) That cautionary note notwithstanding, Scott's mastery of a wealth of primary sources combined with her narrative skill allow her to relate women's organizational activities to the larger context of their evolving and expanding social role.

Scott uses society and association records to show that, since the early days of the Republic, women have organized to achieve goals that seemed to them important. It is clear in retrospect, she says, that such women, constrained by law and custom, and denied access to most of the major institutions by which the society governed itself and created its culture, used voluntary associations to evade some of these constraints and to redefine "women's place" by giving the concept a public dimension. What developed was a complex interconnecting network of women operating in a wholly separate entity within the domain of public affairs. Women were not only contributing to the expansion of American democracy, but were learning to be professionals before the professions were open to them. They learned how to conduct business, carry on meetings, speak in public, and manage money. Women also developed a recognizable female style of professional behavior that relied heavily on cooperation.

The scope of women's activities documented by Scott is staggering. The earliest "female societies" supplemented institutional structures of family, church, and local government by establishing orphan asylums, schools, employment services, homes for wayward girls, libraries, and old ladies' homes. Societies of free black women in the East were among the first to form self-education groups. (Unlike white women, they were also less given to distinguishing between "worthy" and "unworthy" recipients of aid.) The young nation's growing sense of "freedom's ferment," in part fired by the Second Great Awakening, spurred some women to increased activism in the areas of moral reform, temperance, abolition, women's rights, and opposition to prostitution.

The experienced and wide network of women's organizations quickly responded to the crisis of the Civil War. Before the days of K rations, the PX, and a professional medical corps, women of both the Union and the Confederacy provided essential support for their respective military forces in the form of food, clothing, nursing care, and family aid. Scott points out a "bitter irony" in all of this: "if women on both sides had kept closer to their assigned sphere and let the two governments muddle on without their labor, the short war which so many had predicted might indeed have occurred, and nearly everybody would have been better off."

The rapid urbanization that followed the Civil War created new community problems, and women's organizations (increasingly confident as well as national in scope) were among the first to recognize and to begin to deal with these problems. Scott notes that though women did not thereby set out to build what we now call "the welfare state," they did persuade governments to take on many of the responsibilities for human welfare that they themselves originally had assumed. It is impossible, she argues, to imagine American community existence without the institutions and programs put in place by women.

How is it that women were able to engage in so much public activity without encountering significant community opposition? Scott argues that women were able to persist because they were fulfilling the basic cultural expectation that women should be compassionate and nurturing. Their work was considered "municipal housekeeping" (a subset of what has come to be called "maternalist politics"). The largely noncontroversial nature of this "women's work,"—even though it "often transformed the health and appearance of whole towns"—says Scott, also explains its invisibility in history.

Though Scott's focus is not ideological or historiographical debate (which is not insignificant), she makes clear her standpoint. Noting that "the institution of the voluntary association has been available, and used by, people of all political and social persuasions . . . from the Ku Klux Klan to the Green Party," she explicitly chooses to focus on "reform" groups. She holds what she calls "a somewhat old-fashioned view" of the Progressive Era, and gently challenges those who question (deconstruct) women's motives for their benevolent works. Rather than second-guess, Scott prefers examining the surviving records of individual societies to learn more of the consciousness of the women themselves, "a sensibility so different from our own that only a strenuous effort of historical imagination enables us to begin to see the world as they saw it." In fact the very title of her book, taken from a line by Euripides ("Woman is woman's natural ally"), indicates her implicit argument that female associations were on balance intended to be a force for good, rather than an exercise in power that exerted "social control" over the poor and created a middle-class elite.

The book's notes are rich, and Scott, insisting that her work is only a beginning, is generous in suggesting lines of inquiry for future researchers. Her scholarly and readable synthesis provides an essential dimension to any study of American history and should put to rest forever the query, "where were the women?" Though the emergence of professional nursing and the modern hospital are not explicitly discussed, *Natural Allies* provides a broad and essential social context in which to understand these advances and the support they received from reform-minded women. Lastly, one can only marvel once again that the significant role women have played in shaping this society and its institutions has been so overlooked for so long.

Marianne Bankert
Historian and Consultant
American Association of Nurse Anesthetists
1992–93 Fellow of the Wood Library
Museum of Anesthesiology
Park Ridge, Ill.

The Path We Tread: Blacks in Nursing, 1954–1990

By M. Elizabeth Carnegie
(New York: National League for Nursing, Second Edition, 1991)

Because of the popularity of the first edition of *The Path We Tread,* published in 1984, Dr. M. Elizabeth Carnegie updated its contents for the second edition to span the 136 years from 1854 to 1990. The new edition has its own preface but also includes the original preface, in which Carnegie explains her motivation for undertaking the extensive research required. She was concerned about the lack of a "comprehensive history of black nursing," about the brief statements contained in other histories of nursing regarding the contributions made by black nurses to health care, and about the omission from other histories of individuals and events that affected blacks in nursing.

There are significant changes in five of the six chapters, providing evidence of the expanding and important contributions of black nurses to health care and society. Chapter five has not been changed because it contains biographical sketches of the pioneers in nursing, all of whom are deceased.

In the first chapter, Carnegie chose stories of five black women who served in three wars—the Crimean, Civil, and Spanish American—as "illustrations of the contributions made by many in the course of the war." Her concise descriptions of the three wars introduce the accounts of the courageous black women who served as nurses, "most of whom were untrained," and the obstacles they overcame to serve their countries. Unknown to this reviewer was Mary Seacole, a woman from Jamaica, British West Indies, whose request to join Florence Nightingale in the Crimea as a nurse was denied by the British government and also by Nightingale herself. In spite of these rejections, Mary Seacole built and opened with her own money a lodging house on the road between Balaklava and Sebastopol for the comfort of the troops. "On the lower floor was a restaurant and bar; the upper floor was arranged like a hospital ward with her supply of medicines, many of which she concocted herself and used to nurse the sick among the officers." She was eventually honored by the Jamaican government and the British Commonwealth for "saving the lives of countless soldiers wounded during the Crimean War and thousands of others with cholera, yellow fever, malaria, diarrhea."

Chapter 2, titled "The Foundation Is Laid," relates the struggle and courage of individuals and organizations credited with the development of nursing education programs for blacks because "quota systems restricted the admission of black students" when the early schools of nursing were established in the United States. The same restrictions applied to advanced education, as evidenced by the description of two special courses in public health nursing and two in nurse-midwifery established especially for blacks, and the four master's degree programs at historically black institutions.

The humble beginnings of Spellman College as an Atlanta Baptist Female Seminary in 1881 and its decision to establish the first nursing program for blacks in the United States in 1886 provide an example of a nursing school outside of a hospital. As Carnegie noted in the first preface, "All history books credit the University of Minnesota as having established the first nursing program in a University in 1909" and have not credited the School of Medicine at Howard University, Washington, D.C., for admitting seventy-five nursing students in 1893. The nursing program at Howard University was, however, short-lived, because of financial problems and because there was a general consensus "that higher education for women was neither necessary nor practical."

Lists of diploma nursing program for blacks (1886–1982) and of baccalaureate and associate degree programs at historically black schools (1990) provide the location, year established, and, when appropriate, year closed.

"From Dreams to Achievement" is the title of chapter 3, in which the impact of four special projects on the recruitment of blacks and other minorities into nursing is highlighted. Three of the projects were funded by the federal government: the U.S. Cadet Nurse Corps, Breakthrough to Nursing (a project of the National Student Nurses' Association), and the

Ethnic/Minority Fellowship Project administered by the American Nurses' Association (ANA). The fourth was the privately financed Sealantic Project for the Disadvantaged.

In the chapter titled "Struggle for Recognition," the author gives a brief history of more than twenty professional organizations and the leadership roles attained by many black nurses. According to Carnegie, it has been easier for black nurses to participate more fully in some of the newer organizations than it has been for them to attain policy-making positions within the ANA. The emergence of the National Black Nurses' Association in the early 1970s to meet special needs of black nurses and "the health needs of the black community" is recounted, as are the remarkable accomplishments of the National Association of Colored Graduate Nurses (NACGN), which held its final meeting in 1949 after ANA agreed to absorb its functions. One of the better known functions initiated by NACGN in 1936 and undertaken by ANA is the presentation of the Mary Mahoney Award, given for "outstanding contributions in the area of intergroup relations." Known as "America's first trained nurse," Mary Mahoney was one of four students from a class of forty-two to complete the sixteen-month course at the New England Hospital for Women and Children in 1879. All recipients of the award are listed in the appendixes, and their accomplishments are noted throughout the book. Within this chapter are biographies of black nurses who are fellows of the American Academy of Nursing. Carnegie served as Academy president in 1978.

Historical information about the various branches of the military, the Veterans Administration, and the U.S. Public Health Service serves as a backdrop for poignant accounts of black nurses who have distinguished themselves in service to the country.

Carnegie's extensive reference list and bibliography, and the chronology of individual actions and other pivotal events affecting black nursing are valuable, especially to teachers and students of nursing history. The biographies of the identified nurse leaders are a welcome addition to the 1983 publication *Contemporary Minority Leaders in Nursing* (Miller and Mason, 1983).

This book is a well-documented, comprehensive history of black nursing, but it is also much more. Carnegie's interpretation of events about nursing and society in general are an added dimension for anyone engaged in studying or researching the development of professional nursing. The contributions of blacks to nursing and health care, as delineated in *The Path We Tread,* should be incorporated into every history of nursing course. As

Josephine A. Dolan states in the introduction, "Through [Dr. Carnegie's] efforts, a gold mine of information and illustrations not available previously have been vividly portrayed."

MARY D. MUNGER, MSN, RN
Helena, Mont.

References

Miller, Helen, and Ernest Mason. *Contemporary Minority Leaders in Nursing* (Kansas City: American Nurses' Association, 1983).

Private Matters: American Attitudes Toward Childbearing and Infant Nurture in the Urban North, 1800–1869

By Sylvia D. Hoffert
(Urbana: University of Illinois, 1989)

Advice-givers, doomsayers, and well-wishers all contribute to the public discourse that flows freely when the topic is childbirth. A barrage of written information and advice is also offered pregnant women and their families in the form of pamphlets, novels, and journals. In her book *Private Matters: American Attitudes Toward Childbearing and Infant Nurture in the Urban North, 1800–1860,* Sylvia Hoffert has investigated the effects of both spoken and written public discourse on the private attitudes held in the early nineteenth century by upper- and middle-class white women. Using private diaries and letters, and public documents from the era, such as medical journals, texts, health manuals, ladies' journals and religious journals, and novels, Hoffert's study examines the attitudes held by women in five areas: childbearing and pregnancy, childbirth, the recovery period, infant nurture, and infant death.

In the first chapter, "To Abide the Appointed Hour," Hoffert describes women's attitudes toward childbearing and pregnancy. She found women describing this period as one of anxious waiting for the opportunity to give birth. Their ambivalence emerges as the women speak of their sense of well-being, their illness, their dread, and their anticipation.

The second chapter, "To Stand on the Trembling Verge," explores women's attitudes toward childbirth itself. Hoffert finds evidence that birth is a very private experience in the fact that novels regularly pass over the experience with very little description. She found in the private documents evidence of an increasing acceptance of the medical definition of childbirth as an illness. By the 1830s, women regularly used the terms "ill" and "sickness" to describe labor. The medical attention that class distinction afforded then was an important factor in upper-class women's choice of a physician to attend them at their deliveries. Physicians nurtured the stereotype that upper-class women were more delicate than their hardier lower-class sisters and thus were prone to suffer difficult deliveries that required medical intervention. Relief from pain at whatever cost gained greater priority for the upper- and middle-class women as medical intervention became a more readily available and accepted part of medical practice.

The third chapter, "On a Thread Slender and Weak," details women's attitudes toward the recovery period, a time fraught with the deadly dangers of hemorrhage and puerperal fever. Postpartum depression, or "troublesome emotional reactions," also figure prominently in both the private and public documents Hoffert studied. The medical debate between Holmes and Semmelweiss, who implicated the physician as the source of childbed fever, and Charles Meigs, who refused to accept the infectious role played by the doctor in childbed fever, is traced as it affected women's attitudes and choice of birth attendant. Hoffert indicates that the practice of employing "monthly" nurses for the four-week period following delivery seems to have directly paralleled the increasing use of male midwives in the mid to late eighteenth century; she speculates that a possible source of monthly nurses might have been midwives who were increasingly being replaced by physicians in the care of upper-class women.

The fourth chapter, "What To Do with a Baby," details new mothers' overwhelming sense of responsibility and their attitudes toward infant nurture. "Awful" is a word frequently ascribed to the new duties. Friends, relatives, and advice literature was full of "how-to's" and "what-to-do's" for nearly every circumstance; the ideology of motherhood and the particular ways to fulfill that responsibility were spelled out in detail. Breastfeeding was advocated as the only right way of fulfilling the motherly role. Infectious diseases such as cholera posed grave concerns for new mothers. Weaning problems also received much attention.

The fifth chapter, "A Very Peculiar Sorrow," depicts the intense suffering of both fathers and mothers who lost children. Hoffert determines that the declining number of children born in the early nineteenth century, coupled with the cult of motherhood, made death a particularly tragic occurrence. The metaphors used by poets and novelists emphasized the purity and innocence of babies, reinforcing the responsibilities of motherhood and adding guilt to the already bereaved woman.

In conclusion, Hoffert offers the nineteenth-century concern for privacy, the ideology of motherhood, the increasing availability of birth control, geographic mobility, the growth of cities, the rise of publishing industry, the anonymity of urban life, the opportunities for social mobility, the advances in technology and medical knowledge, and the availability of doctors and nurses as factors that altered the context in which middle- and upper-class women gave birth. She sees women changing the rituals of birth and recovery by hiring doctors, which introduced new tensions into the delivery room. No longer were the woman and her female attendants in control; science and its spokesman, the physician, made the decisions. Hoffert also finds, in her study of the private records of the women, that these women found in the maternal role a deep source of fulfillment. The last sentence of the book reads: "During much of their early married lives, the nursery was the one place where they [Northern urban middle- and upper-class women] were subordinate to no one."

An important contribution Hoffert's book makes to the history of childbirth literature is her focus on the *attitudes* of the women, who portray and interpret their birthing experiences in their own words. While the history of childbirth has received significant attention in such works as Wertz and Wertz' several editions of *Lying-In* (the most recent in 1989), Leavitt's *Brought to Bed: Childbearing in America, 1750–1950* (1986), and Sandelowski's *Pain, Pleasure, and American Childbirth: From the Twilight Sleep to the Read Method, 1914–1960* (1984), this book specifically focuses on the experience of childbirth from the woman's point of view. The expressive, often poignant revelations of the concerns and joys of the childbearing women quoted in this work contribute to the reader's understanding of their experience in a highly readable way.

While allowing the women to speak for themselves is a valuable addition to the literature, critic D. Smith admonishes that, "too often, *Private Matters* is marred by a narrow, often literal, reading of source materials" (Smith, 1990). Other critics contend that missing from this work is an integration of current research in social history, women's history, and professional health history of the period (Moldow, 1991). For example, the Popular Health Movement of the 1830s and 1840s, seen by some historians as one of the first major health movements in the United States focused around the beliefs, practices, and concerns of women, is not mentioned in this work that purports to focus on the attitudes of women (Ehrenreich, 1972). In addition, Hoffert's method of interspersing women's personal accounts with fiction, religious, and prescriptive literature is confusing. It blurs the insights that could have been gained had fiction and fact been clearly separated.

Readers of intellectual history will be interested in the development of the ideas about childbirth that Hoffert has provided through her portrayal of the attitudes held by Northern urban upper- and middle-class women between 1800 and 1860. Those concerned with women's history will also find here another source that contributes to the growing body of work that is making women visible in history.

Those who hope to learn about the attitude of childbearing women toward nurses in the early nineteenth century will be disappointed. There are brief references to nurses that cover several areas: employment, training, services, wages, relations with doctors, and dependence of mothers on nurses. Unfortunately, none of these areas is explored in depth. The assumption seems to be that a nurse will be there when needed, but who she is, what she does, and how she affects the health or, in this case, the attitude, of the patient is not explored.

Despite these drawbacks, Hoffert's work brings to light new sources for examining the history of the early nineteenth century. She has provided a useful appendix that details biographical information on the women quoted in her study, and her bibliography of primary sources is extensive. A detailed index provides easy access to specific references in the book.

Sylvia D. Rinker, RN, MS
Assistant Professor
Lynchburg College
Lynchburg, Va.

References

Ehrenreich, B., and D. English. *Witches, Midwives and Nurses: A History of Women Healers* (Old Westbury: The Feminist Press, 1972).
Moldow, G. "Book Review." *American Historical Review* 96 (February 1991): 262.
Smith, D. "Book Review." *Journal of American History* 77 (June 1990): 292.

Always a Sister: The Feminism of Lillian D. Wald

By Doris Groshen Daniels
(New York: The Feminist Press, 1989)

Lillian Wald (1867–1940) is known as the mother of American public health nursing and the founder of New York City's renowned Henry Street

Settlement. This book is the first full-length, feminist biography of Wald to appear, although there has been much written about her by nurses and others, including a 1938 biography by Robert Duffus. Some of her many speeches and letters have been published in several sources, and a play based on her life has been performed and published (Coss, 1989).*

The introduction reveals that "this book is not meant to be a traditional biography of Lillian Wald" (p. 2); the author does not recount Wald's life chronologically. Rather, she deals with her life thematically, "in order to show that her major work as a social reformer was rarely separated from her desire to improve the position of women" (p. 2). Daniels believes that Wald's feminism has been ignored, and this book is meant as a corrective to that belief.

Wald founded the Visiting Nurse Service and the Henry Street Settlement in 1893. Daniels' thesis includes the assertion that these agencies served as the sources of her power and prestige, and that through them she directly contributed to "almost every aspect of the feminist movement" (p. 2).

Partly through an analysis of Wald's personality and temperament (described variously as "conciliatory," "tough-minded," and "circumspect"), Daniels moves through the book describing Wald's privileged childhood in Rochester, her nursing training at New York Hospital, and her now familiar "calling" to visiting nursing in the slums of New York's lower East Side. Chapters 3 and 4 are particularly interesting as she describes "The Education of a Reformer" and "Winning Friends and Influencing Politicos." In example after example, Daniels shows how Wald deserved her reputation as "a person whose heart was always in the right place and was greatly respected because she was loved" (p. 47). The author skillfully weaves in the nursing "sisters" and Wald's commitment to them, as well as her significant contributions to "public health nursing," a term she is credited with originating.

Chapters 5 and 6, titled "A Woman's World" and "A Woman's Mind," represent an exploration of the uniquely female world of Henry Street and of the "new woman" of the early twentieth century. Wald's companions and acquaintances were among many of the prominent female reformers of the

*The Lillian Wald Papers from the holdings of Columbia University's Rare Book and Manuscript Library have now been microfilmed. Their extent (90 reels) attests to Wald's voluminous output of speeches and correspondence—and these are only some of the archival holdings on Wald.

day: Jane Addams, Alice Hamilton, Lavinia Dock, Florence Kelley, Eleanor Roosevelt, to name a few. The character of Wald's relationships with several of these women becomes a focal point for Daniels as she investigates the question of whether Wald was a lesbian. I believe this to be the wrong question to ask: the whole discussion becomes tedious and ultimately meaningless. Blanche Weisen Cook handles the issue of women's relationships with one another in a much more sensitive and productive way in her new book, *Eleanor Roosevelt*.

Nurse historians, public health nurses, and feminist historians will probably constitute the audience for this book. At 154 pages, the book is rather short for a full-length biography, particularly given the extent of Wald's papers, and is more descriptive than analytic. It is clear that Daniels likes her subject and wants to "rescue" Wald from those who believed that she had sold out to her backers and to "the Victorian ideology of her childhood prescribing marriage and motherhood" (p. 154).

Instead of engaging in the women's history debates about feminism after 1920 (see, for example, Cott [1989] and Offen [1988]), Daniels concludes: "Wald worked as hard as she was able for women's rights after 1920" (p. 141). In the concluding pages of the book, she seems to want to excuse Wald and her companions (as if this were necessary) for not being more involved in women's rights. Daniels states, "If the feminist movement declined after 1920, the causes are to be found in the economic conditions and social climate of the nation, not in the behavior of the feminists" (p. 150). A description of Wald's health, losses, and disabilities in the 1920s furthers Daniels's argument that "it wasn't their fault." Surely there is more to the story than this, although perhaps the author wrote the book before the history debates began to rage. Nevertheless, this is a disappointing conclusion to a very useful book that has long been needed.

MERYN STUART, RN, PhD
Assistant Professor, School of Nursing
Adjunct Hannah Professor, History of Medicine, Faculty of Medicine
University of Ottawa
Ontario, Canada

References

Coss, Clare, ed. *Lillian D. Wald: Progressive Activists* (Old Westbury: The Feminist Press, 1989).

Cott, Nancy F. *The Grounding of Modern Feminism* (New Haven and London: Yale University Press, 1987).
Offen, Karen. "Defining Feminism: A Comparative Historical Approach." *Signs* 14 (1988): 119–57 (see also subsequent commentary in *Signs*).

Nurses' Work, The Sacred and The Profane

By Zane Robinson Wolf
(Philadelphia: University of Pennsylvania Press, 1988)

A title like this invites the reader to scan the book just to see what it will say! What one finds is an ethnography describing the work of the staff on a thirty-two-bed medical unit in a large urban hospital in the United States in the 1980s. Following an introductory chapter depicting the physical plant, the pattern of the twenty-four-hour day, and the composition and interactions of the staff, successive chapters focus on postmodern care, medication administration, medical aseptic practices, and the change-of-shift report. The detailed descriptions are written largely in "hospital language" with explanations offered for the lay reader.

In the preface the author states that "nurses' work has both sacred and profane aspects" and that therefore it is "not surprising that a system of rituals exists." She further assumes that the American hospital is a quasi-religious or sacred institution. These remarks led me to anticipate reading a book that would help me to view acute care institutions with "different glasses," as the author's themes were illustrated, explored, and expanded.

The chapter on postmortem care, the longest of the four, actually deals with several phenomena that surround death in an acute care hospital. The author captures the pressures that resource scarcity exerts on the situation. She describes in detail the family interaction and dilemmas as death approaches and/or "Do Not Resuscitate" (DNR) orders are considered. The taxonomy of "almost no code," "slow code," "full code," and the true, urgent effort to resuscitate when death is totally unexpected is amply described and illustrated. Her description of the conflicts produced by the legal need to attempt painful resuscitation in all situations lacking a DNR order, even though nurses recognize that death has gradually approached and become inevitable, is vivid and compelling. Finally, the learning and giving of postmortem care itself, wherein the body is "washed as in morning care," the manifestations of suffering are removed, and nurses "gradually relinquish their tenure of responsibility for the patient," is explored. This chapter was for me the most satisfying and useful in the book.

The chapter on medication administration gives a "snapshot" that is more dated, or perhaps region- or hospital-specific, than descriptions offered in other chapters. Nevertheless, it portrays the immense amount of detail that nurses must attend to in medication administration, the time pressure and need to integrate this task with other duties, the interdependence of nursing with other professions' functions, and the specialized jargon of medications. She points out the almost magical power attributed to medicines and the corresponding lack of acknowledgment of other more interpersonal contributions to healing. She comments on such behaviors as the "ritualistic" three-step check to prevent medication errors, the belief of some nurses that passing medications in a certain pattern prevented errors, and the persistent use of the soufflé cup despite its inadequate size and the availability of unit-dose packaging. Of note, she describes nurses' roles in teaching medical students and new residents how to order medications.

Bathing and management of incontinence were the major focus of the chapter on medical asepsis. The handling of specimens and secretions received some attention, as did the fear of AIDS and herpes zoster. But the major changes that came with the implementation of universal infection control precautions is not intimated. For that reason, this chapter will be useful to future historians. Multiple purposes and meanings of bathing emerged as bathing came variously to be: a time to listen to patients; an opportunity for skin assessment; a support for patient self-esteem; a preparation of the patient for the day; and an indication of respect for the body. The disorganizing effect of late or missing linens in the morning, the ordering effect of the bath-giving on the remainder of the day, and the off-shift rhythm of patient bathing were noted.

In contrast to other activities, the author identifies the change of shift report as an occupational nursing ritual, interpreting its function as suspending time and, to a large extent, activity so that oncoming nurses can begin work with an orderly perspective. The shift report also supports the group's ability to manage difficult aspects of the nursing role. New nurses find it a test of their ability to organize and present facts deemed salient by the unit's nurse culture. For future historians this chapter will provide a perspective on the nursing work culture and perhaps be a date marker for the ever-shifting boundary and overlap of responsibility between nursing and medicine.

My expectation that I would see the world of acute care with "different glasses" was, however, largely unfulfilled. Nowhere did the author describe the distinguishing features of "sacred" and "profane" or provide background on the concepts from cultural anthropology.

The author's definition of ritual, a "patterned symbolic action that refers to the goals and values of a social group," although repeated at significant points in the narrative, is not further developed in the book. Missing from this definition is the rationale or reason for the specific nursing activity. Current nursing behavior that lacks conscious recognition of the reasons for its existence certainly is ripe for the ritualistic label, but the author offers little insight into the reasons behind such activity.

Nursing's "pervasive value" of "doing good and avoiding harm" was cited repeatedly in relation to ritual, but any examination of nursing's definition of "the good" was left unwritten. Elaboration in these areas would not have been necessary for an audience of cultural anthropologists, but it would have greatly increased the value of the work for a nursing audience. The author's vantage point as both "insider" and "outsider" to nursing might have provided a rich interpretation.

As an ethnography, however, *Nurses' Work* certainly passes the test of providing a realistic description of everyday nursing as nurses practice it. This description is important in itself. It will provide historians in 2043 and beyond with an elaborate description of nursing as practiced today in hospitals. (Should the book go to a second edition, it would be helpful if the author identified in the preface the year in which data were gathered). The chapter on postmortem care would be useful for prelicensure students who have little firsthand experience in this area. And for acute care nurses who need a fresh perspective on the significance of their work, the book may provide a starting point for their own individual or group reexamination of the social and human meaning of nursing.

Marilyn E. Flood, RN, PhD
Associate Dean, Academic Program
University of California at San Francisco
San Francisco, Calif.

Civil Wars: Women and the Crisis of Southern Nationalism

By George C. Rable
(Urbana: University of Illinois Press, 1989)

George Rable's *Civil Wars: Women and the Crisis of Southern Nationalism* is a comprehensive work of original research and synthesis that connects three disparate subjects often given cursory attention by historians: the South, women, and the Confederacy (p. ix). In an attempt to answer complex questions about the relationships among gender, class, and race in the sustenance of the southern social order, Rable examines the roles of upper-class women, yeoman women, and poor white women. He provides a sweeping portrayal of southern women within the settings of the antebellum, bellum, and postbellum periods, focusing on how the Civil War in particular affected women. In so doing Rable provides in-depth answers to two underlying questions: (1) "How did white women of various classes assimilate, adjust to, embrace, change, or rebel against their society's definitions of women's place," and (2) "To what extent did the Civil War undermine white women's social identity, their view of themselves, their world?" (ix)

Rable's themes are broad and his archival sources numerous. He sympathetically examines and describes the effects of poverty, hunger, shortages of supplies, and work overload on southern white women during the war, openly acknowledging that a discussion of the role of black women was beyond the scope of this work. Rable excels in providing the reader with diversified accounts of the women's experiences, perceptions, and thoughts. He uses specific illustrations to show how women actively and passively collaborated with men to maintain the existing social order. According to Rable, white women did more to uphold than to undermine the value system of the Old South during both the antebellum and bellum periods.

Rable examines in some depth the thesis of the Civil War as a family crisis. The author is realistic rather than romantic in his description of how the war affected families, noting that the common theme of suffering and the travail of dealing with the ordinary problems of daily living overrode the theme, frequently mentioned by other historians, of expanded opportunities outside of the home. According to Rable, "The war left women with some sense of accomplishment in a world beyond the home, but such memories faded quickly. In later years, most wives and mothers would more clearly recall . . . their families' travail, the shattering of hopes and dreams, and . . . the terror of being left at the mercy of the enemy armies" (p. 153).

The author does, however, explicate the secondary theme of expanded opportunities outside of the home, devoting a chapter to this topic. Included in the chapter "New Women of the Confederacy" is Rable's sketch of Confederate nursing. While not extensive or particularly detailed, this discussion provides the reader with an overview of the commonly acknowledged influential nursing leaders of the South, including Mary Chesnut, Kate Cumming, Phoebe Pember, and Sally Thompkins. In several pages Rable manages to accurately capture the essence of southern women's nursing work during the war, noting the volunteer nature of the work, the hardships the women experienced as a result of shortages in supplies and food, the disorganization of the government's plans for the care of the sick, and the hostility of surgeons to the presence of women in the hospitals during the early years of the war.

Of specific interest to scholars of Civil War nursing history is Rable's success in placing the nursing activities of women within the larger social and political setting. He discusses nursing in the context of the demands made on women as a result of the reality of the war, the social forces, and the prevailing ideology regarding women's place in nineteenth-century southern society. Rable observes that because of various family demands, the roles of women during the war were diverse. Many women stayed home and managed plantations and farms. Others operated lumber mills and ferries, clerked in stores, taught in schools, and worked as postmistresses. Not every woman volunteered to provide nursing care to the soldiers. Rable also notes how the prevailing social ideology affected women who nursed the sick. He discusses the ideological contradiction in the prevalent belief that women were supposed to preserve their gentle nature but at the same time take whatever steps necessary to care for the wounded and sick. In this light, Rable calls attention to the fact that "the emphasis on volunteers meant that women working in hospitals would do so temporarily and not neglect their domestic duties" (p. 121). According to the author, "in the tradition of antebellum ladies . . . some volunteers and nurses viewed hospital work as poor relief, a part of their customary obligation to uplift the downtrodden" (p. 123). The view that charitable activities were a natural extension of women's moral superiority and religious sensibility was predominant in nineteenth-century society. Rable points out that "when women nursed the sick, wounded and dying soldiers, they also nurtured conventional ideas about their own place and character" (p. 121).

Of significance to nurse historians is the insight Rable provides into the tensions between plantation mistresses, yeoman women, and poor white women. The author asserts: "The mixture of benevolence, professionalism and necessity made it difficult for women of widely varying backgrounds to work together harmoniously. Indeed, the familiar stories of altruistic angels of mercy reveal little about the complex lives of Confederate nurses, especially the refugee women and soldier's wives whose primary motive for working in hospitals may well have been money" (p. 123). I would agree that there was much conflict among the women who nursed the sick. However, I am not sure to which "familiar altruistic stories" Rable is referring when he makes this comment or whether he is stating a popular assumption. In my reading of accounts by women who nursed in the Confederacy, I found not altruistic stories, but detailed, depressing documentation of the stresses, strains, hardships, and conflicts that these women experienced (Keeling, 1989). Rable therefore should be applauded for his accuracy, perceptive interpretation, and realism in his accounts of nursing in the South.

In conclusion, by portraying a panoramic view of women in the South, Rable cannot focus on a particular social class of women, as Clinton does in *Plantation Mistress* (1982), nor can he provide an in-depth account of one specific group of women that cut across class lines, such as those women who nursed the sick during the war. However, Rable's ability to present with some cohesiveness and analysis the findings of his exhaustive research far outweighs these weaknesses. The author has made a major contribution to the field of southern women's history. His book should be read by historians and nursing scholars interested in southern women, nursing, and the Civil War.

Arlene W. Keeling, PhD, RN
Assistant Professor
Associate Director, The Center for Nursing Historical Inquiry
School of Nursing
University of Virginia
Charlottesville, Va.

References

Clinton, C. *The Plantation Mistress: Women's World in the Old South* (New York: Pantheon Books, 1982).

Keeling, A. "Supporting the Cause: Nursing Activities of Southern Women during the Civil War" (Paper presented at the Sixth Annual American Association for History of Nursing Conference, Baltimore, Maryland, 1989).

Images of Nurses: Perspectives from History, Art, and Literature

Ed. by Anne Hudson Jones
(Philadelphia: University of Pennsylvania Press, 1988)

At a time when nurses are concerned with their public image, the title of this book seems to promise a good read. And indeed it is, although not quite in the way that I had anticipated. Perhaps as a nurse familiar with the work of many fine historians who are also nurses, I was a bit disappointed by the roster of authors. I suppose it would be professioncentric (if there is yet such a word in the politically correct vocabulary) to assume that nurses have a special perspective from which to view the images of nurses. Although one might argue for the objective perspective that other disciplines would bring to the task, my disappointment lingered long enough for me to mentally list possible nurse historians who could have been included among the authors. I consoled myself by imaging that lurking behind one of the essayists might be a nurse friend or relative, and I was further comforted by the recognition of several of the authors as collaborators in projects with nurses and by acknowledgments within the essays of input from nurse colleagues.

Each of the book's contributors carries impressive credentials in women's history, nursing history, literature, research on images, women's studies, art history, architectural history, American studies, and/or women's issues. The book grew out of a research project exploring images of nurses from the perspective of a variety of disciplines. The authors involved had an opportunity to discuss their essays and reshape them, based on critiques from one another. Interestingly, although the editor acknowledges that "nurses and humanists—most of them feminist scholars—worked across disciplinary lines . . . to begin a dialogue that has enriched the subsequently revised essays," none of the nurses appears in more than a footnote.

The book is divided into three parts. In part one, Natalie Boymel Kampen explores images of nurses in the visual arts from prehistoric times to the seventeenth century. The second author, Rima D. Apple, prepared an essay on the photographic images of hospital nurses in the late nineteenth and early twentieth centuries. Karen Kingsley focuses on the architecture of nursing, that is, on nurses' residences and schools of nursing as they existed in the late nineteenth century and were later transformed in the twentieth century.

The four chapters in the second part of the book are devoted to images of nursing and nurses in literature. Leslie Fiedler explores the images in fiction and popular culture. Kathryn Montgomery Hunter's chapter, "Nurses: The Satiric Image and the Translocated Ideal," is designed to complement Fiedler's images. Short stories of the twentieth century provide content for Barbara Melosh's analysis in "'A Special Relationship': Nurses and Patients in Twentieth Century Short Stories," and Joanne Trautmann Banks, in "Voltaries of Life: Patrick White's Round-the-Clock Nurses," has chosen one novel to illustrate her thesis.

The final section is devoted to an exploration and analysis of the interaction between images and social issues in the twentieth-century United States. Darlene Clark Hine's historical images of black nurses is followed by an essay by Janet Muff about sexism and socialization in nursing. The editor closes the book with an analysis of Hollywood's image of Florence Nightingale.

Kampen's opening essay is an admirable attempt to review images of women as health care workers in the Greek and Roman art of the fifth century B.C. to the fourth A.D., in the art of the fifteenth and sixteenth centuries, and in seventeenth-century Flanders art. Kampen has chosen pieces representative of these periods to illustrate her essay. Apart from omitting any mention of Fabiola (built the first general hospital in Rome in A.D. 390) and Hygeia (goddess of health maintenance or, as Dolan says, "the embodiment of nurses") as context from Greek mythology for the later portrayals, this is a fascinating treatment of an interesting subject. To be fair to the author, the famous J. J. Henner portrait of Fabiola obviously does not date from the periods covered in the chapter.

The photographs in Apple's chapter are a fascinating look at nurses' hospital work in the latter nineteenth century. Of necessity, in an essay and not a book-length treatment of this subject, the author, rather than attempting to cover the subject comprehensively, has chosen sixteen representational photos. Institutional histories would provide many photographs to be included in a larger work, as would the archives of municipal libraries, such as the New York Public Library and the Boston Public Library. In addition, the National Library of Medicine has a significant collection of nursing photographs.

Perhaps the most fascinating chapter in this book is that on the architecture of nursing, probably because it is a perspective least familiar to me. I have often mused on the cottage hospital and nurses' home architecture of New England, and on the stately oriental rug–bedecked living rooms found in their gracious nurses' residences. Kingsley has more than fulfilled the promise of her title. This well-written essay is accompanied by site plans, architectural drawings, photographs, and models. Perhaps my only criticism, more a comment, is that she does not mention the contribution of Minnie Goodnow, a noted historian of nursing, but also—germane to this topic—a draftsperson and hospital architect.

The four chapters on nurses and nursing in American literature left me with several queries. While the author's decision to illustrate nursing with a single novel is interesting, the rich store of literary allusions to nursing is thereby left untapped. Why only the brief mention of the work of the

Kalisches? Why not Louisa May Alcott as an example, not perhaps as opposed to but in addition to Walt Whitman? Surely Melosh is aware of Mary Roberts Rinehart (a trained nurse) and her many short stories with nurse characters and heroes. In the final essay, Banks defends the choice of a single illustrative novel with the statement that "the most practical book about nursing I know . . . is *The Eye of the Storm*." Even after many pages of detailed description of the novel, however, I am not convinced of its universalness. You may be.

Darlene Hine's carefully researched essay on black nurses reflects her immersion in an important story, to date only partially told. I would like rationale for her choice of stories, but this omission does not detract from the value of the selection nor from its usefulness in illustrating the images of black nurses during sixty years of service.

I wish that Muff would explore in more depth the images perpetuated by schools of nursing entrance requirements and their training programs in her analysis of socialization and sexism. A discussion of Ashley's 1980 work, published in *Advances in Nursing Science,* which called into question our somewhat thoughtless adoption of a male model of professionalism, would also be fitting to this topic. An essay, however, cannot be an exhaustive treatise, and this piece is among the best and most thought-provoking available on these topics.

The editor closes the book with an essay on the reduction of Florence Nightingale by Hollywood from a powerful, brilliant woman to "a popular and palatable image for mass consumption . . . thus idealizing her and diminishing her at the same time." Jones makes a sound case for her thesis that such "images can become more influential than the historical reality on which they are based." Hers is a fitting essay to close a well-written book, crammed with new and exciting perspectives from a wide variety of disciplines.

Still a good read? I'll give it a resounding yes. And to whom might it appeal? Certainly to all nurses, but also to historians and others interested in nurses and nursing, or in portrayals of women, especially professional women, in history, art, and literature.

JOELLEN W. HAWKINS, RNC, PhD, FAAN
Professor
School of Nursing
Boston College
Boston, Mass.

Worse Than the Disease: Pitfalls of Medical Progress

By Diana B. Dutton
(New York: Cambridge University Press, 1988)

Worse Than the Disease is the result of a multidisciplinary research project at Stanford University. It is a well-written, stimulating, and carefully referenced work in which the author and her two contributors, Thomas A. Preston and Nancy E. Pfund, explore the influences of medical innovations on social, ethical, and economic dilemmas in American society. Dutton makes a compelling case for the general public's active participation in solving the problems engendered by technological innovations. She does this gradually, presenting the evolution of four cases in the second half of the twentieth century.

Highlighted cases are the development and use of synthetic estrogen or diethylstilbestrol (DES), of the artificial heart, of the Swine Flu immunization program, and of genetic engineering. The author scrutinizes each case by examining violations of ethical principles, especially of autonomy and justice. She contends that the initial introductory phase of an innovation fashions its future agendas. Expert opinion provided in the beginning of such a technological advance, she argues, creates a point of view that may become difficult to change later.

Over an extended time period, for example, scientists and physicians failed to adequately question their initial lack of concern regarding the consequences of DES therapy. Originally touted as a medication to prevent miscarriages, the wonder drug was prescribed for purposes for which it had not been carefully evaluated. The administration of DES resulted in harmful effects, such as increased risk of breast cancer in DES mothers and in DES daughters because of transplacental carcinogenesis and vaginal adenocarcinoma. In the initial phases of DES use, the medical community was "caught up in a tide of pro DES sentiment" (p. 59). In this case, the Federal Food and Drug Administration was both part of the problem and the solution, failing to act until it had no alternative.

The artificial heart, the second case presented, proved incapable of prolonging a high quality of life among recipients. Patients who received the device suffered strokes and many discomforts. The artificial heart illustrated the capacity of rank commercialism to spoil a technological advantage for patients, since true medical advances were not realized in its use. The Swine Flu immunization program, as another case, was shaped by society's fear and government politics. For a while, doubts of a few experts were voiced but ignored and, because of the seriousness of the side effects of the vaccine, the program was eventually considered the Vietnam of the Public Health Service. The feared epidemic never arrived and fatalities from Guillain-Barré syndrome forced officials to more carefully weigh the risks and the benefits of immunization programs. Dutton cautions experts to use worst-case thinking in the future. Finally, the amazing biotechnical displays that have already brought the world feats of genetic engineering have "concealed" the fears of some scientists that future discoveries of molecular biology may have detrimental effects on the environment. Here too, the author raises ethical concerns expressed by some groups about the potential hazards of genetic engineering on human reproductive cells.

Throughout the book, Dutton emphasizes the power and unknown implications of advances in modern science and medicine and suggests that it may be impossible to weigh thoroughly the risks to society. She points out that as innovations are adopted, the political interests of the federal government and the pecuniary interests of the corporate world complicate the picture. This is especially true when harmful results follow. Furthermore, the former devotion of academic scientists to science for the sake of knowledge alone has been gradually derailed by business contributions to highly productive universities. Scientists have lost their innocence and have become business partners. One of the author's greatest fears seems to be that the prompt and dispassionate disclosures of scientific findings to society will be eradicated as scientific knowledge increasingly becomes "private property that can be owned and traded for profit" (p. 209). Dutton warns of society's limited ability to predict the future effects of innovations, and notes that medical innovations, such as the artificial heart, have consumed many health care dollars and temporarily extended the life of a few rather than many Americans. She asserts that social values serve as a powerful analytic structure by which to study the effects of technology and to guide the development and implementation of social policies.

The author has produced a scholarly work presenting her arguments cogently and astutely. When reaching the end of the text, the reader will not be as surprised at the author's recommendations for the careful evaluation of future innovations. Historians interested in twentieth-century history of medicine will find the weaving of theoretical arguments and supporting facts convincing. Historians of medicine and nursing will appreciate the book, since it raises many issues for historical research, among them the history of covert rationing of health care services.

While written for a general audience, the book appeals in particular to those concerned with the threat of technologies to individual and societal life, and to the world's ecological balance. Dutton reiterates her belief that prospective and concurrent public participation in biomedical policy decisions will assist scientists and practitioners in keeping the consequences of these innovations in clearer focus and decrease the influence of the self-serving agendas of special interest groups. Defining the public as those "professionals in fields unrelated to the innovation in question, and representative of public interest organizations" (p. 322), the author values the vision of the lay public, whose perspective may be fresher than those of experts directly involved in the developing technologies.

Dutton delineates the elements of policy discussions, and acknowledges that costs, risks, and benefits factors do not apply to all issues associated with biomedical innovations. Her advice reminds the reader to remember the 1960s when the citizens of the United States demanded that their concerns be taken seriously by national decision-makers; the views of experts, she suggests, should always be challenged. Finally, her warnings of a national bias toward medical intervention rather than toward prevention should be carefully heeded.

Zane Robinson Wolf, PhD, RN, FAAN
Professor, La Salle University
Associate Director of Nursing for Research, Albert Einstein Medical Center
Philadelphia, Pa.

SUBJECT INDEX

GUIDELINES FOR CONTRIBUTORS

To facilitate publication of your contribution, we ask that you follow these guidelines in preparing your manuscript. For solicited articles, length guidelines and submission deadlines will be specified in the solicitation letter. Unsolicited submissions are welcome at any time and will be acknowledged promptly; manuscript length should be appropriate to the topic of the submission.

The entire manuscript (including notes, quoted or set-off text, and references) must be typed fully double spaced. Single-spaced typescripts will be returned to the author for retyping. All typescripts must be prepared with a typewriter or letter-quality computer printer. Draft-quality dot-matrix printouts will not be accepted for publication. Margins of at least one inch on all sides must be maintained. Please submit the original (ribbon) copy of the typescript and three photocopies. All pages, including reference pages, should be numbered consecutively. Please omit any author identification lines on manuscript pages to facilitate blind review.

The cover page for your article must include the following: article title (no more than two parts: title and subtitle); full names of author(s) as meant to appear in print; the address, telephone number, and fax number for the corresponding author; brief acknowledgments of support or assistance; and at least six key words or phrases to be used in subject indexing.

Up to three levels of text headings may be used in your typescript; these must be differentiated clearly in your manuscript by distinct and consistent indentations and capitalization. For questions of note style, please follow the guidelines for numbered endnotes in *The Chicago Manual of Style* (13th edition). All notes must be double-spaced and typed separately from the text (i.e., placed at the end of the article rather than as footnotes). Reference lists should be used solely to provide bibliographic data for sources cited in the text.

Tables must be typed double-spaced, each on a separate sheet, and must be accompanied by a title and/or legend. Figures (line drawings, photographs, etc.) must be submitted as black-and-white camera-ready glossy prints. All drawings, graphs, and charts must be professional-quality. Illustrations prepared with computerized graphic programs will not be accepted unless they are indistinguishable from professional-quality artwork drawn by a graphic artist. Glossy prints must be labeled on the back with the name of the article, author(s), and figure number. Photographs must be accompanied by an appropriate credit line (name of photographer, archive, or collection). Captions or legends for all figures must be typed double-spaced and provided on a sheet separate from the figures themselves. Be sure to make explicit reference to each figure and table within the text, but attach all tables and figures to the end of the typescript.

If more than 500 words of text are quoted from a scholarly book or 250 words from a scholarly article, or if a table or figure has been previously published, the article manuscript must be accompanied by written permission from the copyright owner (who is not necessarily the author of the quote, table, or figure). It is the responsibility of the author to determine who owns the copyright and to submit the appropriate permission letters. Final acceptance of the manuscript will be withheld until all necessary permission letters are received.

All correspondence concerning your submission should be sent to: Joan E. Lynaugh, Editor, *Nursing History Review,* University of Pennsylvania, 420 Guardian Drive, Room 307, Philadelphia, Pa. 19104-6096. Phone: (215) 898-4502; Fax: (215) 573-2168.

American Association for the History of Nursing

You are invited to join the American Association for the History of Nursing, whose mission is to preserve, promote, and disseminate information about the history and heritage of the nursing profession.

What are the purposes of the AAHN?

• Stimulate national and international interest in the history of nursing, promote collaboration among its supporters, and encourage research in the history of nursing.

• Promote the development of centers for the preservation and use of materials of historical importance to nursing.

• Serve as a resource for information related to nursing history.

• Produce and distribute materials related to the history and heritage of the nursing profession.

What are the benefits of AAHN membership?

• Receive the official AAHN journal *Nursing History Review*, published annually in January and devoted to the history of nursing and health care:

Long neglected, the history of nursing has recently become the focus of a considerable amount of attention. Over the past decade, developments in the history of medicine, the history of women—particularly of women's work—and nursing itself have resulted in a new recognition of the importance of the subject.

As the official journal of the American Association for the History of Nursing, Nursing History Review *enables those interested in nursing and health care history to trace new and developing work in the field. The* Review *publishes significant scholarly work in all aspects of nursing history as well as reviews of recent books and updates on national and international activities in health care history.*

• Establish linkages with others who are ardent about the history of the nursing profession.

• Receive the AAHN quarterly *Bulletin*, which keeps you informed about calls for abstracts, fellowship and grant opportunities, conferences, book releases, and other news related to the history of nursing and the AAHN.

• Attend annual AAHN conferences where refereed papers and posters on a wide range of history of nursing subjects are presented, a book mart of historical reference material is conducted, and an auction consisting mainly of nursing memorabilia is held.

• Extend your professional insight through dialogues with colleagues.

• Learn how to compete for the annual prestigious Lavinia L. Dock and Teresa E. Christy awards, which recognize exemplary historical research and writing related to nursing history.